RESEARCH PROGRESS ON EPINEPHRINE

RESEARCH PROGRESS ON EPINEPHRINE

ARNOLD G. LAWSON AND ROGER I. GORMAN
EDITORS

Nova Biomedical Books
New York

For permission to use material from this book please contact us:
Telephone 631-231-7269; Fax 631-231-8175
Web Site: http://www.novapublishers.com

Library of Congress Cataloging-in-Publication Data

Research progress on epinephrine / Arnold G. Lawson and Roger I. Goman, editor.
p. ; cm.
Includes bibliographical references and index.
ISBN 978-1-60456-443-3(hardcover)
1. Adrenaline. I. Lawson,Arnold G. II. Gorman, Roger I.
[DLMN: 1. Epinephrine.2.Research. WK 725 R432 2008]
QP572.A27R47 2008
612.4'5—dc22

2008006486

Published by Nova Science Publishers, Inc. ≈ New York

Contents

Preface

This new book is devoted to new research on epinephrine (INN) sometimes spelled "epinephrin" or "adrenalin" respectively, which is a hormone when carried in the blood and a neurotransmitter when it is released across a neuronal synapse. It is a catecholamine, a sympathomimetic monoamine derived from the amino acids phenylalanine and tyrosine. When secreted into the bloodstream, it rapidly prepares the body for action in emergency situations. The hormone boosts the supply of oxygen and glucose to the brain and muscles, while suppressing other non-emergency bodily processes (digestion in particular).

It increases heart rate and stroke volume, dilates the pupils, and constricts arterioles in the skin and gut while dilating arterioles in skeletal muscles. It elevates the blood sugar level by increasing catalysis of glycogen to glucose in the liver, and at the same time begins the breakdown of lipids in fat cells. Like some other stress hormones, epinephrine has a suppressive effect on the immune system.

Although epinephrine does not have any psychoactive effects, stress or arousal also releases norepinephrine in the brain. Norepinephrine has similar actions in the body, but is also psychoactive.

Epinephrine is used as a drug to treat cardiac arrest and other cardiac dysrhythmias resulting in diminished or absent cardiac output; its action is to increase peripheral resistance via á1-adrenoceptor vasoconstriction, so that blood is shunted to the body's core, and the â1-adrenoceptor response which is increased cardiac rate and output (the speed and pronouncement of heart beats). This beneficial action comes with a significant negative consequcnce—increased cardiac irritability—which may lead to additional complications immediately following an otherwise successful resuscitation. Alternatives to this treatment include vasopressin, a powerful antidiuretic which also increases peripheral vascular resistance leading to blood shunting via vasoconstriction, but without the attendant increase in myocardial irritability.

Short Communication A - Background of the Study: Between 2002 and 2004, the Japanese National Committee on the Prehospital Emergency Medical Services (EMS) system discussed whether Emergency Life-Saving Technicians (ELSTs), who, up to that time, were prohibited from administering drugs, should be allowed to administer resuscitative drugs such as epinephrine for out-of-hospital cardiopulmonary resuscitation (CPR). This issue created considerable debate among emergency care experts in Japan since, at that time, there was little evidence that epinephrine contributes to survival from out-of-hospital cardiac arrest.

In 2003, the authors undertook a prospective study to provide information for the discussion of whether resuscitative drugs should be introduced into the Japanese EMS system, in which ELSTs play an important role.

Conceptual Framework of the Study: Rather than focusing on evaluation of resuscitative drugs themselves in the prehospital setting, we compared the results of use of such drugs in two different EMS systems.

Study Design: Areas served by doctor-manned ambulances, where out-of-hospital CPR was performed with resuscitative drugs (making up an experimental area), and areas served by ELST-manned ambulances, where resuscitative drugs were not administered outside the hospital (making up a reference area), were included in the study. The sequence of emergency procedures performed in the experimental area was divided into three phases: phase I included administration of epinephrine; phase II started with the use of other resuscitative drugs, lidocaine or atropine; and phase III started with administration of any other drug. Outcomes, i.e., resuscitation rates and 1-month survival rates, were determined, and differences between the experimental area and reference area were analyzed.

Results of the Study: For non-traumatic cardiac arrest, phase I outcomes were better in the experimental area than in the reference area. Outcomes through phase II were significantly better in the experimental area than in the reference area.

Change in the EMS System: In April 2006, Japan adopted an EMS system allowing ELSTs to administer epinephrine only. This choice was made not only because of data indicating the effectiveness of epinephrine, but also in consideration of other factors including methods of on-line medical control and risk of accidents.

Short Communication B - Ibopamine is a dopamine analogue and it is hydrolysed to epinine by the esterases in the aqueous humor. It stimulates alpha-adrenergic receptors and D1-dopaminergic receptors in the eye. Adrenergic stimulation is responsible for the non-cycloplegic mydriatic effect, while the D1-dopaminergic activity increases the aqueous humor production. Ibopamine is useful as a mydriatic before and after surgical procedures. Its main uses are: provocative test in glaucoma; treatment of ocular hypotony; evaluation of the outflow pathways of the aqueous humor. Ibopamine test is positive in 92% of patients affected by primary open-angle glaucoma (POAG), while it is negative in healthy eyes. It is useful to detect an outflow impairement in relatives of glaucomatous patients.

Chapter I - Within- and between-session environmental habituation were examined in infant rats on postnatal days 14 and 15 in an open field. Using a computerized animal tracking system, rats showed decreases in the total distance traveled (m) and overall average speed (m/s) across 6 30-sec time blocks each day and from day 1 to day 2 of testing. Although the literature is inconclusive regarding the ontogeny of environmental habituation, these results provide clear evidence of both within-session and between-session habituation. On postnatal day 16, animals were returned to the open field with 2 identical objects for novel object recognition training. Animals were either tested immediately after training or were given a subcutaneous injection of saline or .01 mg/kg of epinephrine, followed by testing 2-hrs later. For testing, animals were placed into the open field with one familiar and one novel object, and the number of object explorations and the time spent exploring each object were recorded by the animal tracking system. From these measures the absolute mean preference for novelty and relative percent preference for novelty were computed. Only the relative percent preference for novelty based on the time spent exploring each object revealed significant differences among the groups. Post-hoc pair-wise comparisons indicated that saline animals tested 2-hrs after training performed significantly worse than epinephrine animals and worse than those tested immediately after training. This indicates a rapid rate of forgetting for object recognition memory which is effectively attenuated with post-training epinephrine.

Chapter II - Cardiac diseases are frequent causes of morbidity and mortality all over the world which signify a major priority field in medical research. However, a significant improvement has been made during the last decades in diagnosis and therapy of cardiac diseases, which invites the need for better understanding of their pathophysiological basis. Many neurohormoral changes occur as a consequence of the hemodynamic alternations in cardiac diseases, of which increased sympathetic nervous modulation is likely to be detrimental to cardiac diseases. Epinephrine (Epi) has the sophisticated cross-talk with some physiological substances, the critical involvement in the cardiac regulation in both health and diseases, and the adapted effect to stress. Although about ninety percent of major origins for Epi are from adrenal medulla, much less is known about extra-adrenal tissues. The origin of such extra-adrenal epinephrine stores has been explained by neuronal uptake, neuronal synthesis, synthesis by extra-adrenal chromaffin cells and neuroendocrine cells. Phenylethanolamine N-methyltransferase (PNMT), an enzyme involved in Epi synthesis, is widely distributed not only in adrenal gland but also in other organs. In the heart, the PNMT is localized not mainly in intrinsic cardiac adrenergic system, but might also be in cardiomyocytes, suggesting the presence of Epi system in the heart. Hence the development of knowledge for Epi in the heart would extend further our knowledge in understanding cardiac diseases.

Chapter III - Epinephrine is a natural catecholamine. It is a potent stimulator of both α - and β-adrenergic receptors. Its expression of action might be local that acts in the field of body administered or systematic while administered via one of the intravenous or parenteral routes. The expression of action for epinephrine administered systematically depends on the part of the body and type of adrenergic receptors involved. With its α-1 adrenergic properties on skin and subcutaneous tissue, epinephrine is an extremely potent vasoconstrictor.

Epinephrine, being a potent vasoconstrictor, is used ubiquitously in plastic surgery where concentrations as low as 1:200,000 to 1:400,000 provide sufficient vasoconstriction to decrease bleeding at the operative field.

Recent studies described a sustained epinephrine release model in vivo. Using microspheres, which is a part of a drug delivery system, a sustained epinephrine release is achieved. These studies have shown that sustained epinephrine release caused a vascular augmentation in vivo. This augmentation resulted in favorable morphometric, like increase in vessel wall diameter, number of vessels and dilatation, and hemodynamic alterations.

The data extracted from the studies bodes great potential in surgery. Sustained epinephrine release might be applied in bleeding control of operative fields that lasts more than a few hours such as in burn surgeries or highly vascularized operative fields such as scalp and face. On the other hand the ability of intentionally augmenting the vascular network in vivo without surgery holds great potential for flap surgery. As a final, it is shown that high epinephrine applied to a soft tissue is causing tissue necrosis. High concentrations of epinephrine release via the aforementioned drug delivery system might be applied to decrease a tumor volume by causing tissue necrosis. In this case, high concentrations of epinephrine would be applied locally and functioning as a 'chemical killer' for tumor cells.

Chapter IV - Epinephrine is one substance among several others that contributes to platelet activation. Platelet activation is crucial for normal haemostasis but can also be deleterious in the setting of thrombosis. The activating effect of epinephrine on platelets is achieved through α_2-adrenergic receptors (α_2-ARs). Present on platelets are also inhibitory β-adrenergic receptors. However, the importance of these latter receptors for *in vivo* platelet function is unknown. Signalling from the α_2-ARs go through the G_z-protein. A result of this is lowered levels of intracellular cAMP but the signalling pathways stimulated by epinephrine are far more complex than this. Consequently, this is a research area that needs more investigation. It is also important to consider activation with epinephrine in the context of other platelet activators, since this is the case *in vivo*. Epinephrine is known to develop synergistic effects with platelet activators such as thrombin, lysophosphatidic acid (LPA), platelet-activating factor (PAF) and serotonin. It has actually been emphasized that epinephrine cannot function on its own on platelets but needs to cooperate with other activators. Furthermore, synergistic platelet adhesion and aggregation induced *in vitro* by epinephrine combined with LPA is dependent on secretion of adenosine-di-phosphate (ADP). Thus, in these cases two additional activators are needed besides epinephrine to achieve platelet activation. The importance of epinephrine for thrombus formation *in vivo* is not totally clear but several studies support a connection between increased levels of epinephrine and cardiovascular events. Increased levels of epinephrine might synergize with other platelet activators released after atherosclerotic plaque rupture resulting in accelerated thrombosis.

Chapter V - Epinephrine is a prime mover in the "fight or flight" response. Epinephrine elevates heart rate, reduces blood flow to the skin, increases the production of sweat, and increases vigilances. Epinephrine widens the smaller bronchioles in the lungs, dilates the pupils of the eyes and its action on the liver raises blood-sugar levels by stimulating glucose production. In adipose tissue epinephrine raises blood fatty-acid levels. These effects on the cardiovascular system could perhaps play an important role in the onset and maintenance of hypertension.

Epinephrine accounts for 80%, while norepinephrine accounts for 20% of the total hormone secreted from the adrenal medulla. Several studies have reported that epinephrine can augment neurogenic vasoconstriction, while other investigators have shown that urinary or plasma epinephrine levels are correlated with blood pressure. There is not general agreement on this latter point. In several epidemiological studies of either cross-sectional or a longitudinal design, our findings have demonstrated no relationships between plasma epinephrine levels and blood pressure or heart rate.

The "epinephrine hypothesis" proposes that circulating epinephrine is taken up by sympathetic nerves, thereby promoting norepinephrine release during sympathetic nervous system stimulation. It is suggested that binding of co-released epinephrine to pre-synaptic β-adrenoceptors augments exocytotic release of norepinephrine and contribute to high blood pressure (hypertension). Thus, the "epinephrine hypothesis" might explain how adrenomedullary hormonal system activity can contribute to the development of essential hypertension by augmenting sympathoneuroral norepinephrine release.

There is evidence that the sympathetic nerves of hypertensive patients release epinephrine as a co-transmitter. In this review, results will be presented which suggest that epinephrine is synthesized in situ in sympathetic nerve endings via the action of phenylethanolamine-N-methyltransferase (PNMT), which is induced by chronic mental stress exposure. Accordingly, this represents a biomarker of chronic mental stress, rather than a specific mechanism of hypertension, as suggested by the "epinephrine hypothesis".

Chapter VI - It has been discussed that acute and slow-growing lesions involve different patterns of reorganization. Regarding the anatomical relationships between the motor cortex, the pons, and the cerebellum, the authors evaluated the effects of an acute lesion (cortical ablation) and a Fe2Cl-induced slow-growing lesion in order to study their effects on the pontine and cerebellar norepinephrine (NE) contents, since this neurotransmitter has been involved in the recovery of the lost functions.

Sixty-five male wistar rats (280-320 g) were allocated into six groups: sham-operated A (SA; n=11), sham-operated B (SB), injured by cortical ablation (CA), injured by cortical ablation and recovering (CAR), injured by Fe2Cl intraparenchimal injection in the motor cortex (Fe), and injured by the same procedure and recovering (FeR). Their footprints were obtained 24 hours before the surgery as a basal record. Then, 35 rats were operated upon and the right hindlimb motor area (MCx) was aspirated in the CA (N=6) and CAR (n=12) groups, while all the procedures without aspiration were performed in the SA (n=11) group. Then, the footprints were recorded every 6 hours for 48 hours. In the remaining subjects, a cannula directed to the MCx was surgically placed in the SB (n=16), Fe (n=5), and FeR (n=16) groups. Thus, artificial cerebrospinal fluid (CSF, 5μl) was injected in free-moving conditions in the SB animals, while CSF containing Fe2Cl (50 mM) was injected into the Fe and FeR groups. Footprints were recorded for 15 days. At the end of the recording periods, the rats were sacrificed by decapitation and the left and right sides of the pons and cerebella were removed. NE contents were analyzed by HPLC, and the remaining encephallus was used in order to delimitate the respective lesions. Comparisons were performed using the Mann-Withney U test (p=0.05).

Results showed that recovery in ablated animals was faster than in Fe2Cl injured rats. The authors also observed a pontine NE increase in CA animals and a NE decrease in Fe rats, turning to normal levels in recovering rats. Cerebellar NE was unaltered in CA group, decreased in Fe animals and unaltered in FeR animals.

These results demonstrate that the NEergic mechanisms involved in the recovery after brain injury depends on the kind of the lesion. This suggests the need to evaluate the nature of the injury in order to develop clinical strategies in the treatment in humans.

Chapter VII - Epinephrine in the heart is believed to be taken up mainly from the circulation by sympathetic nerve endings. However, at least three additional sources of epinephrine in the mammalian heart have been suggested to date: 1. Intrinsic ganglion neurons displaying phenylethanolamine N-methyltransferase (PNMT)-immunoreactivity, enzyme decisive in epinephrine synthesis; 2. Intrinsic cardiac adrenergic cells distinct from adrenergic neurons; 3. Myocardial cells containing inducible PNMT or nonspecific N-methyltransferase.

The aim of the study presented in this chapter was to evaluate epinephrine and norepinephrine release from the atria and left ventricles of rats subjected to neonatal chemical sympathectomy by guanethidine in comparison to age-matched controls.

At the age of 8 months, the heart atria or left ventricles were dissected, sliced, pooled and transferred into 12 parallelly perfused perfusion chambers. Tissues were superfused with oxygenated Krebs-Henseleit (KH) solution. After 40 min equilibration period, basal release of catecholamines was measured and then norepinephrine or epinephrine outflows were stimulated by depolarization with 50 mmol/l KCl in the superfusion fluid. Norepinephrine and epinephrine concentrations in superfusates were determined using radioimmunoassay ultrasensitive diagnostic kits. The effects of tyramine (10^{-6} mol/l), desipramine (10^{-7} mol/l), and dibutyryl cAMP (10^{-4} mol/l) were tested in the atria and left ventricles. In addition, resting heart rate and blood pressure were measured bimonthly and epinephrine and norepinephrine concentrations were determined in the heart compartments of control and guanethidine-treated animals at the ages of 4 and 8 months.

At the age of 8 months, the tissue concentrations of norepinephrine in the denervated atria and left ventricles did not exceed 20% and 10% of the control values, respectively. In contrast, epinephrine concentrations did not significantly differ between guanethidine- and vehicle-treated preparations.

Basal release of norepinephrine from the control samples was significantly enhanced by depolarization (high KCl), dibutyryl cAMP, tyramine and desipramine. Stimulated norepinephrine release (high KCl) was significantly higher in the presence of tyramine, desipramine and dibutyryl cAMP. Basal release of norepinephrine from the sympathectomized heart was significantly lower than that from the control preparations and it was enhanced by tyramine, desipramine and cAMP. In contrast, epinephrine release from the denervated atria and ventricles was not affected by depolarization, tyramine and desipramine, but it was significantly increased by dibutyryl cAMP.

The authors' results provide further evidence of epinephrine signaling system independent of the sympathetic innervation in the mammalian heart. Epinephrine release from non-neuronal sources might help to maintain cardiac functions in the absence of sympathetic innervation.

In: Research Progress on Epinephrine
Editors: A. G. Lawson and R. I. Gorman, pp. 1-11
ISBN: 978-1-60456-443-3

Short Communication A

Effectiveness of Out-of-hospital Cardiopulmonary Resuscitation with Resuscitative Drugs such as Epinephrine

Kenji Ohshige*
Department of Public Health, Yokohama City University School of Medicine
3-9 Fukuura, Kanazawa-ku, Yokohama 236-0004, Japan

Abstract

Background of the Study

Between 2002 and 2004, the Japanese National Committee on the Prehospital Emergency Medical Services (EMS) system discussed whether Emergency Life-Saving Technicians (ELSTs), who, up to that time, were prohibited from administering drugs, should be allowed to administer resuscitative drugs such as epinephrine for out-of-hospital cardiopulmonary resuscitation (CPR). This issue created considerable debate among emergency care experts in Japan since, at that time, there was little evidence that epinephrine contributes to survival from out-of-hospital cardiac arrest.

In 2003, we undertook a prospective study to provide information for the discussion of whether resuscitative drugs should be introduced into the Japanese EMS system, in which ELSTs play an important role.

* Tel: +81-(0)45-787-7610; Fax: +81-(0)45-787-7609; E-mail: kenoh@med.yokohama-cu.ac.jp

Conceptual Framework of the Study

Rather than focusing on evaluation of resuscitative drugs themselves in the prehospital setting, we compared the results of use of such drugs in two different EMS systems.

Study Design

Areas served by doctor-manned ambulances, where out-of-hospital CPR was performed with resuscitative drugs (making up an experimental area), and areas served by ELST-manned ambulances, where resuscitative drugs were not administered outside the hospital (making up a reference area), were included in the study. The sequence of emergency procedures performed in the experimental area was divided into three phases: phase I included administration of epinephrine; phase II started with the use of other resuscitative drugs, lidocaine or atropine; and phase III started with administration of any other drug. Outcomes, i.e., resuscitation rates and 1-month survival rates, were determined, and differences between the experimental area and reference area were analyzed.

Results of the Study

For non-traumatic cardiac arrest, phase I outcomes were better in the experimental area than in the reference area. Outcomes through phase II were significantly better in the experimental area than in the reference area.

Change in the EMS System

In April 2006, Japan adopted an EMS system allowing ELSTs to administer epinephrine only. This choice was made not only because of data indicating the effectiveness of epinephrine, but also in consideration of other factors including methods of on-line medical control and risk of accidents.

Introduction

Background of the Study

Between 2002 and 2004, the Japanese National Committee on the Prehospital Emergency Medical Services (EMS) system established by the Ministry of Health, Labour and Welfare, and the Fire and Disaster Management Agency of the Ministry of Internal Affairs and Communications, discussed whether Emergency Life-Saving Technicians (ELSTs), who up to that time were prohibited from administering drugs, should be allowed to administer resuscitative drugs such as epinephrine for out-of-hospital cardiopulmonary resuscitation

(CPR). Cardiac arrest that occurs outside the hospital setting requires early CPR and early defibrillation [1-7]. However, despite recommendations by the American Heart Association [1] and the European Resuscitation Council [2] to use epinephrine for cardiac arrest, there existed almost no valid reports concerning the use of epinephrine during out-of-hospital emergency care for patients suffering cardiac arrest [8-12]. In fact, there was no clear evidence of the effectiveness of epinephrine for cardiac arrest in any setting. This could be because epinephrine was administered for cardiac arrest universally and customarily before the concept of evidence-based medicine was established.

It was under these circumstances that specialists engaged in a heated debate over whether to permit ELSTs to administer epinephrine or other medications in cases of out-of-hospital cardiac arrest, perplexing the investigative committee. Consequently, a study was launched regarding the effectiveness of resuscitative drugs when administered by ELSTs. That investigation focused on two scenarios: prehospital administration of epinephrine alone and prehospital administration of three medications: epinephrine, lidocaine, and atropine.

EMS in Japan

In Japan, local governments provide 24-hour EMS as a public service. Anyone can use an ambulance free of charge by making a phone call to '119.' Most local governments use a one-tier system, with basic life support (BLS) ambulances staffed by ELSTs, who are trained to treat patients with cardiac arrest but, until recently, have been prohibited from administering any drugs. Several regions, in addition, have their own two-tier system: BLS ambulances and doctor-manned ambulances. Doctor-manned ambulances provide prehospital advanced life support, including administration of the necessary drugs.

Methods

Conceptual Framework of the Study

A simple analysis of the relationship between drug use and clinical results can lead to erroneous conclusions. For example, if there is a tendency to administer many more medications to individuals who are difficult to resuscitate than to individuals who are easily resuscitated, use of medications can appear to be related to a decreased survival rate. Conversely, if there is a tendency to refrain from drug administration for individuals for whom resuscitation is not probable, the positive effect of medications on survival can be exaggerated. Decisions regarding whether or not to administer medications fall within the realm of medical judgment and can bias any analysis. A proper, unbiased study required that we test the effects of prehospital use of resuscitative drugs for individuals suffering cardiac arrest. We had to find a way to determine whether such drugs should be used for CPR in the prehospital setting, particularly by ELSTs. A randomized-controlled trial (RCT) would have been the best way to answer this question. However, an RCT in which some patients were given resuscitative drugs and others were not would not have been ethically feasible. We considered dividing a large region into zones and allowing some ELSTs to use medications and forming a conclusion based on the results. However, with the regulations in place at that time, this would have been very complicated. Another option might have been to restrict doctors' use of medications so that only target drugs were evaluated. However, although the use of other drugs can mask the effect of the target drugs, it would not have been ethically feasible to restrict use of other drugs.

It was under these considerations and constraints that we chose to use a rather unorthodox study method. Rather than focusing on evaluation of resuscitative drugs themselves in the prehospital setting, we compared the results of use of such drugs in two different EMS systems.

Study Design

The study, due to legal and ethical restrictions, was conducted under the existing EMS system. That is, we studied one area (experimental area) where doctors in doctor-manned ambulances use medications during prehospital CPR for individuals suffering cardiac arrest, and we studied another area (reference area) where ELSTs respond and no medication is used during prehospital CPR for individuals suffering cardiac arrest. Outcomes in the two areas were compared.

Study Target

The study targeted witnessed cardiac arrests occurring outside the hospital. Four areas served by doctor-manned ambulances were selected and together made up the experimental area. Four other areas matching the experimental areas in terms of area, population size, proportion of the population aged 65 years and older, and number of cases of cardiac arrest were selected and together made up to reference area. The reference area operated a one-tier system, with ELST-staffed BLS ambulances.

The prehospital CPR performed with medications in the study was intended to simulate an EMS system in which resuscitative drugs can be used for CPR. The intention was to determine whether the resuscitation rate and 1-month survival rate would improve under such a system and not to evaluate the validity of the drug administration itself. This was because, as long as attempts at resuscitation continued, resuscitative drugs were administered after arrival at the hospital in the reference area.

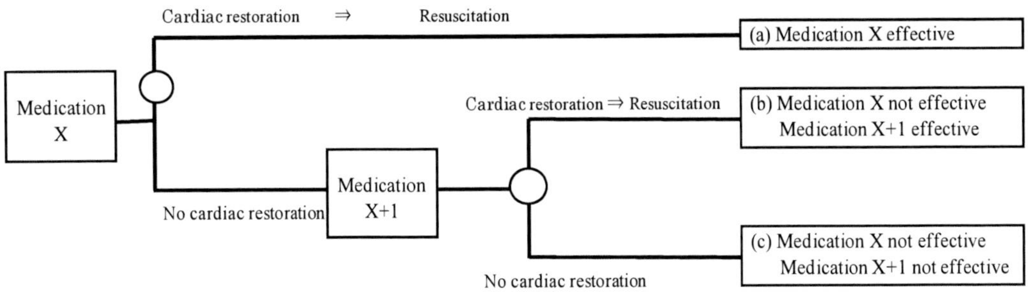

Figure 1. Action tree used to determine whether medication was effective.
Medication X was considered effective only in cases in which it alone was effective (a).

Doctor-Manned Ambulance Action Tree

The sequence of life saving procedures performed in the doctor-manned ambulances was divided into three phases. Phase I included tracheal intubation, defibrillation, cannulation of an intravenous line, and administration of epinephrine. Phase II started with the use of the other resuscitative drugs, lidocaine and atropine. Phase III started with administration any other drug and included all other treatment activities, including those performed after arrival at the hospital.

The action tree for assessing the effectiveness of the medication is presented as a flow chart in Figure 1. When restoration was achieved due to medication X and the patient arrived at the hospital in a resuscitated state, medication X was considered effective (a). If, following the administration of medication X, the patient died despite administration of other medications (medication X+1), medication X was considered ineffective (c). If administration of medication X alone did not produce resuscitation, but addition of another medication produced resuscitation, effectiveness of medication X could not be completely ruled out. However, for the sake of the study, medication X was considered ineffective in this case (b). Thus, it is possible that the effectiveness of drug administration was underestimated. A general overview of the doctor-manned ambulance action tree is reported elsewhere [13].

Effectiveness of Drug Administration and Policy Making

Potential resuscitation patterns are shown in Figure 2. Results were compared against these patterns, and recommendations were made to the National Committee on the Prehospital EMS system on the basis of the pattern that best fit the study results. When the resuscitation rate remains unchanged (pattern A) despite administration of epinephrine alone or the three drugs, prehospital medical procedure dictates that it is not necessary to proceed with drug administration. When the resuscitation rate is increased by administration of the three medications (pattern B), choosing sole administration of epinephrine is not possible. So a choice is made between continuing the present system and administering the three medications. When the resuscitation rate is increasing by epinephrine administration and administration of all three drugs does not change the resuscitation rate (pattern C), administering the three medications must be rejected. A choice is made to continue under the present system or to administer epinephrine alone. When the resuscitation rate is increasing by epinephrine administration and increased further by administration of the three drugs (pattern D), a rational choice between continuing under the current system, sole administration of epinephrine, and administration of the three medications is required. Other factors, such as safety, were considered in the decision-making process. Other patterns were used to illustrate the effectiveness of drug administration, but these four patterns were considered the base upon which policy was decided.

Results

Cases of Cardiac Arrest

During a 7-month study period, there were 162 witnessed cardiac arrests (100 men, 62 women) to which a doctor-manned ambulance responded (experimental area). Forty-one of these were classified as traumatic cardiac arrests, 120 of these were classified as non-traumatic cardiac arrest, and 1 was undetermined. During the same period, there were 272 witnessed cardiac arrests (169 men, 103 women) to which an ELST-manned ambulance responded (reference area). Forty-four of these were classified as traumatic cardiac arrests, 222 were classified as non-traumatic, and 6 were undetermined.

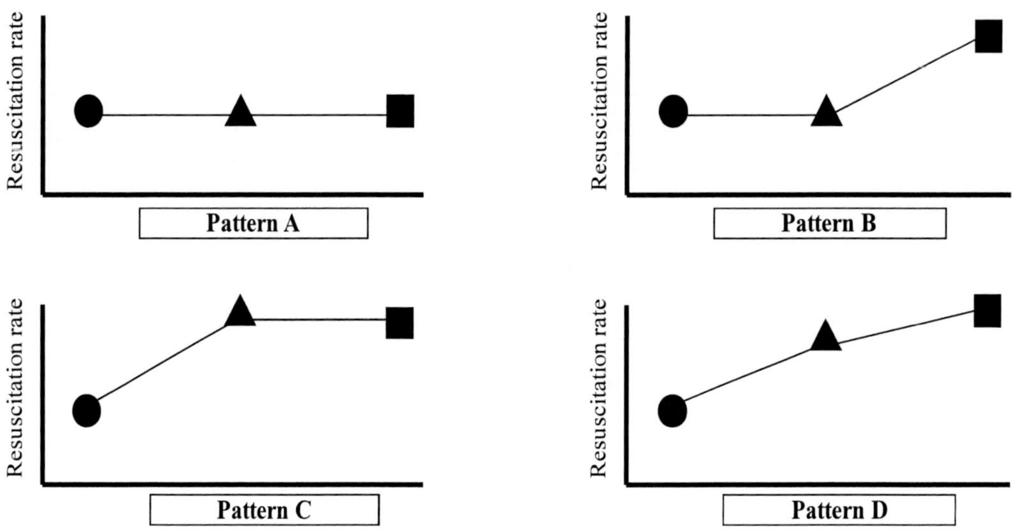

Figure 2. Graph-based patterns of effective drug administration.

Resuscitation rate when ● no drug was administered (current system), ▲ only epinephrine was administered, or ■ three drugs were administered (epinephrine, atropine, lidocaine).

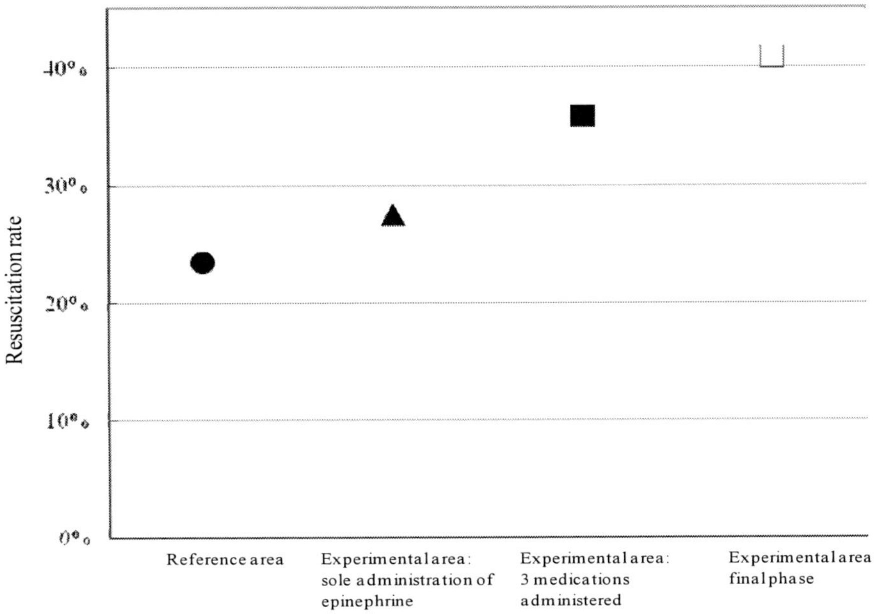

Figure 3. Resuscitation rate for cases of non-traumatic cardiac arrest.
The reference group consisted of cases responded to by ELSTs, while the experimental group consisted of cases responded to by the doctor-manned ambulance.

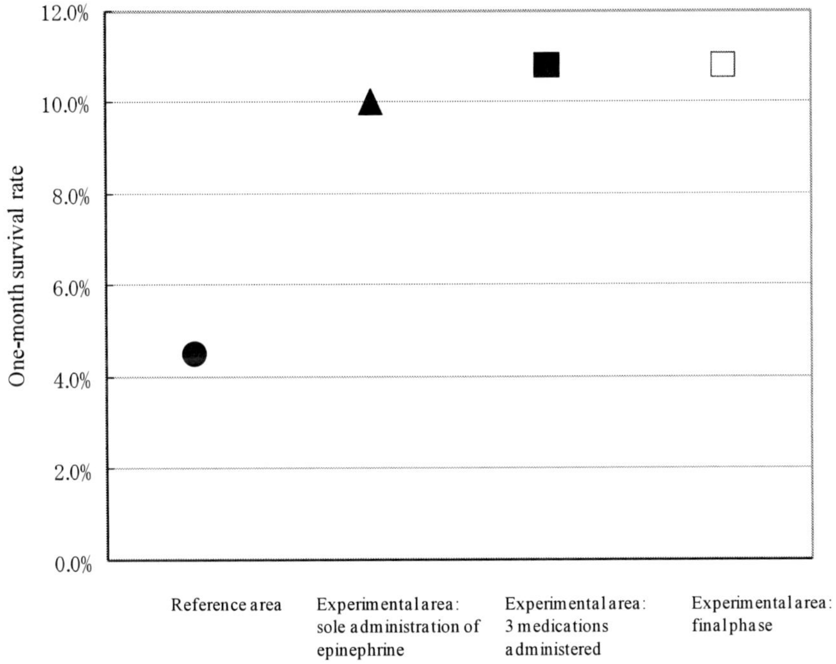

Figure 4. One-month survival rate for cases of non-traumatic cardiopulmonary arrest.
The reference group consisted of cases responded to by ELSTs, while the experimental group consisted of cases responded to by the doctor-manned ambulance.

Resuscitation and 1-month Survival Rates for Patients with Traumatic Cardiac Arrest

A total of 11 patients from the experimental area who suffered traumatic cardiac arrest were resuscitated (resuscitation rate, 26.8%), and 14 patients from the reference area who suffered cardiac arrest were resuscitated (resuscitation rate, 31.8%). Although the rate was higher in the reference area, the difference did not reach statistical significance (P = 0.614). The 1-month survival rate for patients with traumatic cardiac arrest was 9.8% (4 patients) in the experimental area and 2.7% (1 patient) in the reference area, so, unlike the resuscitation rate, the 1-month survival rate was higher in the experimental area than in the reference areas, although the difference was not statistically significant (P = 0.192).

Resuscitation and 1-month Survival Rates for Patients with Non-Traumatic Cardiac Arrest

Forty-nine patients from the experimental area who suffered non-traumatic cardiac arrest were resuscitated (resuscitation rate, 40.8%), and 52 patients from the reference areas who suffered non-traumatic cardiac arrest were resuscitated (resuscitation rate, 24.4%). The rate was significantly higher in the experimental area (P = 0.001). The 1-month survival rate for patients with non-traumatic cardiac arrest was 10.8% (13 patients) in the experimental area, and 4.5% (10 patients) in the reference area. The rate was significantly higher in the experimental area (P = 0.027).

The relation between drug administration and the resuscitation rate in cases of non-traumatic cardiac arrest is illustrated in Figure 3. The resuscitation rate increased from that in the reference area to that in phase I in the experimental area, in which patients were given epinephrine alone, to that in phase II in the experimental area, in which patients were given the three medications, to that in phase III in the experimental area. It became clear that the resuscitation rate improved as options were added in terms of drug administration. The relation between drug administration and the 1-month survival rate in cases of non-traumatic cardiac arrest is shown in Figure 4. It became clear that the 1-month survival rate was greatly increased with sole administration of epinephrine in the experimental area, and that it was somewhat increased with administration of the three medications.

Discussion

There are three principal concerns pertaining to the study. The first is that there may be a discrepancy between the performance standard of doctors in the doctor manned ambulances and ELSTs in ELST-manned ambulances. In other words, compared to the onboard doctor's sole task of providing early resuscitation in the doctor-manned ambulance, the ELST had the combined task of providing early resuscitation and timely patient transport. This difference must be taken into account in evaluating the study results. The resuscitation rate and 1-month survival rate were taken as outcome measures. Resuscitation was defined as a "return of spontaneous circulation when arriving at the hospital, resulting in admission to the intensive care unit (ICU)." In other words, patients whose heartbeat was restored for a period but stopped again before being admission were not considered resuscitated. The second concern was the possibility that there would be a bias in terms of the degree of medical judgment involved in administering medication. Consequently, drugs had to be administered according to guidelines, necessitating the creation of an action protocol. This protocol, based on a rational procedure appropriate for emergency medical situations, took the form of an action tree that allowed for easy analysis. This was an application of decision tree analysis method [14,15]. The third concern appeared during analysis, when analysis was performed using the action tree. It is possible that the effectiveness of drug administration was underestimated. This concern was detailed in the section called Doctor-Manned Ambulance Action Tree.

In this investigation, for cases of non-traumatic cardiac arrest, the administration of epinephrine alone, the administration of three medications, and the administration of the three medications in combination with other medications (by doctors in the doctor-manned ambulances), in that order, resulted in incremental increase in the resuscitation rate. The results were similar to pattern D in Figure 2. Thus, when the resuscitation rates are looked at to determine policy, the best policy would be widespread use of doctor-manned ambulances. Until doctor-manned ambulances can be realized, it would be prudent to allow ELSTs to perform prehospital CPR using the three medications, i.e., epinephrine, lidocaine, and atropine. However, currently, the cost of training ELSTs, the method of online medical control, and the risk of accidents complicate use of the three drugs by ELSTs, so the next best choice would be to allow ELSTs to perform CPR using epinephrine.

Prehospital use of medications by ELSTs represents not only a shift in medical care ELSTs are allowed to provide but also a shift in ELST performance standard, i.e., a shift from "early patient transport" to "early cardiac restoration." There are benefits and drawbacks associated with each task, so a change in ELST performance criteria must be regarded as an extremely important consideration. Results of our study do not identify a suitable balance for how much "early transport" should be sacrificed when trying to achieve "early cardiac restoration."

Conclusion

Our study showed a progressive increase in both the resuscitation rate and 1-month survival rate when no medication was used, when only epinephrine was used, and when three medications were used. It was suggested that prehospital administration of medication by ELSTs would be effective for patients with non-traumatic cardiac arrest. A proper balance between "early patient transport" and "early cardiac restoration" and between medical effectiveness and safety is important.

In April 2006, based on the data obtained from this study, Japan adopted an EMS system in which ELSTs can administer only epinephrine. This choice was made not only because of data indicating the effectiveness of epinephrine, but also other factors including methods of on-line medical control and risk of accidents [16].

References

[1] Guidelines for cardiopulmonary resuscitation and emergency cardiac care. Emergency Cardiac Care Committee and Subcommittees, American Heart Association. Part III. Adult advanced cardiac life support. *JAMA* 1992;268:2199-241.

[2] The 1998 European Resuscitation Council guidelines for adult advanced life support. Advanced Life Support Working Group of the European Resuscitation Council. *BMJ* 1998;316:1863-9.

[3] Cummins RO, Ornato JP, Thies WH, Pepe PE. Improving survival from sudden cardiac arrest: the "chain of survival" concept. A statement for health professionals from the Advanced Cardiac Life Support Subcommittee and the Emergency Cardiac Care Committee, American Heart Association. *Circulation* 1991;83:1832-47.

[4] Kowalski R, Thompson BM, Horwitz L, Stueven H, Aprahamian C, Darin JC. Bystander CPR in prehospital coarse ventricular fibrillation. *Ann Emerg Med* 1984;13:1016-20.

[5] Cummins RO, Eisenberg MS. Prehospital cardiopulmonary resuscitation. Is it effective? *JAMA* 1985;253:2408-12.

[6] Mashiko K, Otsuka T, Shimazaki S, Kohama A, Kamishima G, Katsurada K et al. An outcome study of out-of-hospital cardiac arrest using the Utstein template-- a Japanese experience. *Resuscitation* 2002;55:241-6.

[7] De Maio VJ, Stiell IG, Wells GA, Spaite DW; Ontario Prehospital Advanced Life Support Study Group. Optimal defibrillation response intervals for maximum out-of-hospital cardiac arrest survival rates. *Ann Emerg Med* 2003;42:242-50.

[8] Holmberg M, Holmberg S, Herlitz J. Low chance of survival among patients requiring adrenaline (epinephrine) or intubation after out-of-hospital cardiac arrest in Sweden. *Resuscitation* 2002;54:37-45.

[9] Tang W, Weil MH, Sun S, Noc M, Yang L, Gazmuri RJ. Epinephrine increases the severity of postresuscitation myocardial dysfunction. *Circulation* 1995;92:3089-93.

[10] Callaham M, Madsen CD, Barton CW, Saunders CE, Pointer J. A randomized clinical trial of high-dose epinephrine and norepinephrine vs standard-dose epinephrine in prehospital cardiac arrest. *JAMA* 1992;268:2667-72.

[11] Herlitz J, Ekström L, Wennerblom B, Axelsson Å, Bång A, Holmberg S. Adrenaline in out-of-hospital ventricular fibrillation. Does it make any difference? *Resuscitation* 1995;29:195-201.

[12] Woodhouse SP, Cox S, Boyd P, Case C, Weber M. High dose and standard dose adrenaline do not alter survival, compared with placebo, in cardiac arrest. *Resuscitation* 1995;30:243-9.

[13] Ohshige K, Shimazaki S, Hirasawa H, Nakamura M, Kin H, Fujii C,et al. Evaluation of out-of-hospital cardiopulmonary resuscitation with resuscitative drugs: a prospective comparative study in Japan. *Resuscitation* 2005;66:53-61.

[14] Jones JM. Decision analysis using spreadsheets. *European Journal of Operational Research* 1986;26:385-400.

[15] Dowie R, Campbell H, Donohoe R, Clarke P. 'Event tree' analysis of out-of hospital cardiac arrest data: confirming the importance of bystander CPR. *Resuscitation* 2003;56:173-81.

[16] Ohshige K. Effectiveness of resuscitative drugs in out-of-hospital emergency care. *Journal of Emergency Medical Services (Japan)* 2005;13:12-6. (in Japanese)

In: Research Progress on Epinephrine
Editors: A. G. Lawson and R. I. Gorman, pp. 13-23
ISBN: 978-1-60456-443-3

Short Communication B

Up-to-date on Ibopamine, a New Alpha-adrenergic and D1 Dopaminergic Drug

Italo Giuffre*
Medical School- University of Roma "Tor Vergata", Roma, Italy

Abstract

Ibopamine is a dopamine analogue and it is hydrolysed to epinine by the esterases in the aqueous humor. It stimulates alpha-adrenergic receptors and D1-dopaminergic receptors in the eye. Adrenergic stimulation is responsible for the non-cycloplegic mydriatic effect, while the D1-dopaminergic activity increases the aqueous humor production. Ibopamine is useful as a mydriatic before and after surgical procedures. Its main uses are: provocative test in glaucoma; treatment of ocular hypotony; evaluation of the outflow pathways of the aqueous humor. Ibopamine test is positive in 92% of patients affected by primary open-angle glaucoma (POAG), while it is negative in healthy eyes. It is useful to detect an outflow impairement in relatives of glaucomatous patients.

Keywords: Ibopamine, dopaminergic drugs, non-cycloplegic mydriatic, glaucoma, diagnostic test, ocular hypotony

Introduction

Dopamine is a typical multireceptorial agent which has effects on the cardiovascular system: it increases cardiac output, diuresis and renal excretion of sodium. From dopamine an orally administered compound, ibopamine (3,4 dyisobutyrrilester of N-methyl-dopamine) was

* Address: Via Seneca, 34, 00136 Roma – Italy; Ph./Fax: ++39-0635341166; E-mail: italogiuffre@libero.it

identified and chemically synthesised in 1986 (Figure 1). It is a prodrug of epinine. It has positive inotropic effects: it improves cardiac function and is effective in the treatment of congestive heart failure. In 1986 Virno et al. discovered the ocular pharmacological characteristics of topically administered ibopamine: the α-adrenergic and D1 dopaminergic activities [1,2,3]. Ibopamine, instilled at 2% concentration, has the following effect in the eye:

- Non-cycloplegic mydriatic effect to examine fundus oculi (α-adrenergic activity);
- Pre- and post-operative mydriatic activity;
- Stimulation of aqueous humor production (D1 dopaminergic activity);
- Provocative test in glaucoma;
- Pharmacological test to evaluate the aqueous humor outflow system in relatives of glaucomatous patients;
- Treatment of ocular hypotony.

Both concentrations (1% and 2%) ibopamine were recently tested but they have similar ability to rise IOP (at least 3 mmHg to be considered positive) with a sensitivity of 84.6% and specificity of 73.3% [4].

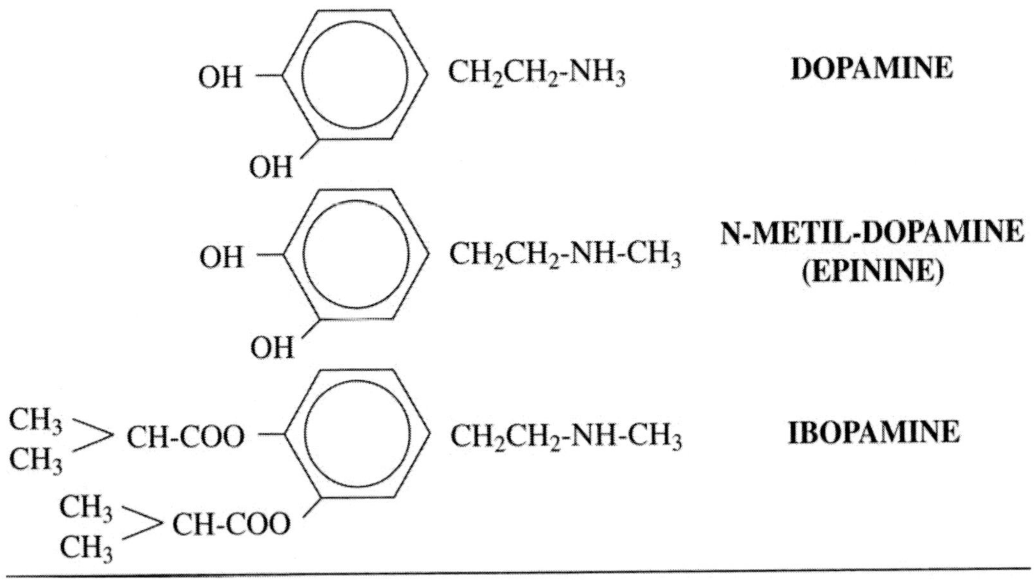

Figure 1.

Pharmacokinetics

In the conjunctival sac, ibopamine is hydrolysed to epinine by the esterases of the aqueous humor and ocular tissues. The epinine is the active component of the molecule: the half-life of ibopamine in the aqueous humor is short (about 2 minutes) [5,6] and epinine precedes the mydriatic effect. After the instillation of ibopamine, only epinine can be found in the aqueous humor [5].

Pharmacodynamics

When hydrolysed to epinine, ibopamine stimulates the α-adrenergic and D1 dopaminergic receptors. Its mydriatic effect is due to the stimulation of the α-adrenergic receptors of the dilating muscle of the pupil. Since ibopamine has no effect on the ciliary muscle, the ibopamine-induced mydriasis is not accompanied by cycloplegia. The mydriatic effect is due to an α-adrenergic stimulation and mydriasis can be antagonized and reversed by pre-treatment by α-blocking agents (such as thymoxamine and dapiprazole). The D1 dopaminergic activity of the drug was shown to increase aqueous humor production and intraocular pressure (IOP) in primary open-angle glaucoma (POAG) patients [7].

Toxicology

Ibopamine has low toxicity both at systemic and local levels. LD_{50} is 2056 mg/Kg, 4930 mg/Kg and 1786 mg/Kg in mice, rats and guinea pigs respectively. Ibopamine is well tolerated without any significant change to the haematological and behavioral parameters (unpublished toxicological studies). 2% ibopamine eye drops showed that ibopamine is well tolerated at local level, without systemic side-effects and tachyphylaxis phenomena. One drop of 2% ibopamine contains 1 mg of the compound, while the oral dosage is higher than 400 mg/day.

Clinical Use

Non-cycloplegic Mydriatic Activity

In the diagnostics, such as binocular indirect examination of fundus oculi with scleral indentation, fluorescein and indocyanine angiography and in the laser treatment of retinal lesions, a locally applied drug such as ibopamine can induce a fast, short-lasting (2-3 hours), maximal mydriasis without cycloplegic effects or local and/or systemic side-effects. The mydriatic effect of ibopamine can be prolonged if repeatedly administered (every 30 minutes). Ibopamine-induced mydriasis can be reversed by local application of α-blockers (such as thymoxamine and dapiprazole). Ibopamine can substitute phenylephrine in association with tropicamide and/or cyclopentolate to avoid the typical discomfort of cycloplegia mostly in adult patients. 2% ibopamine is effective in inducing preoperative mydriasis, without effects on the cardiovascular system. During the postoperative period, also after trabeculectomy, ibopamine can induce a fast and short-lasting mydriasis to induce pupil dilatation and to maintain the filtering bleb.

Stimulation of Aqueous Humor Production by D1 Dopaminergic Activity

Pathophysiology of IOP

2% ibopamine eye drops increases IOP only in patients suffering from POAG. Ibopamine is very useful in different areas, such as:

- Physiological studies on IOP;
- Evaluation of trabecular outflow pathways (pressure-dependent outflow);
- Treatment of ocular hypotony.

Ibopamine increases IOP in about 92% of eyes with POAG; the hypertensive effect is dose-dependent and, after multiple administrations, does not cause tachyphylaxis (Figure 2 [8,9,10,11]. Its sensitivity is 84,6% and its specificity is 73.3% [4]. In normal eyes, 2% ibopamine does not significantly affect IOP, with a mild hypotensive effect (1-2 mmHg) (Figure 2). IOP in POAG patients increases by a maximum value of 10-11 mmHg within 45 minutes from the instillation and lasts about 180 minutes [12,13,14,15]. Two drops of 2% ibopamine have been instilled 5 minutes apart, and IOP was measured 45 minutes after the first instillation. Some graphics show that, pupillary diameter being equal, only ibopamine, compared to 10% phenylephrine eye drops, is able to induce an IOP increase, due to its peculiar D1 dopaminergic effect on aqueous humor production (Figure 3). These α-adrenergic and D1 dopaminergic effects take place without any clinically significant systemic or local side-effects (Figures 4,5,6,7,8,9).

The ibopamine provocative test shows a statistically significant correlation with the highest intraocular pressure in the diurnal tension curve in glaucoma patients [16].

Mechanism of Action

Several studies were performed to assess the following issues:

- Identification of the responsible receptor (agonist and antagonist);
- Evaluation of the change in the aqueous humor dynamics;
- Evaluation of ibopamine effects when the outflow system was experimentally impaired.

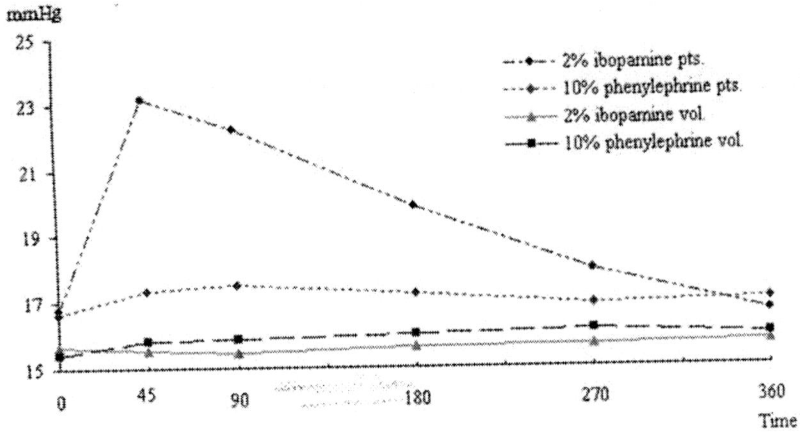

	Maximum increase	Area under the curve
Ibo pts. vs. Ibo vol.	p = 0.0001	p = 0.0001
Ibo pts. vs. Phn pts.	p = 0.0001	p = 0.0001
Ibo vol. vs. Phn vol.	p = n.s.	p = 0.01
Phn pts. vs. Phn vol.	p = n.s.	p = n.s.

Figure 2. Intraocular pressure.

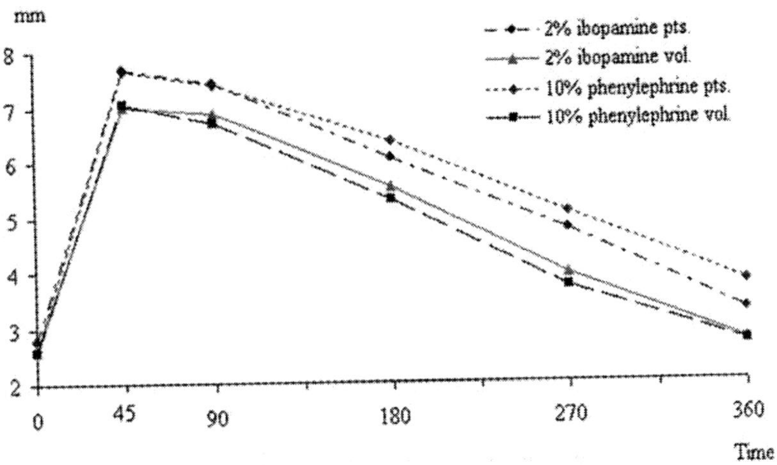

	Maximum increase	Area Under the Curve
Ibo pts. vs. Ibo vol.	p = n.s.	p = n.s.
Ibo pts. vs. Phn pts.	p = n.s.	p < 0.05
Ibo vol. vs. Phn vol.	p = n.s.	p = n.s.
Phn pts. vs. Phn vol.	p = n.s.	p = 0.0002

Figure 3. Pupillary diameter.

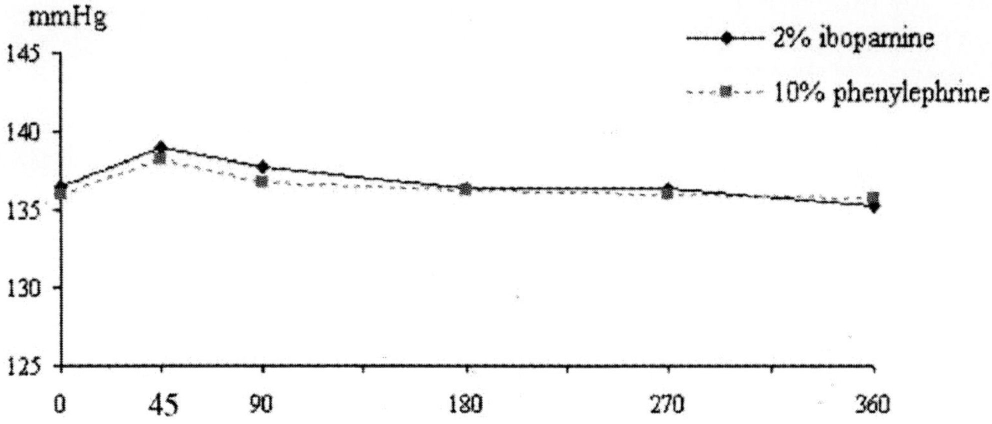

Figure 4. Glaucomatous patients - Systolic blood pressure.

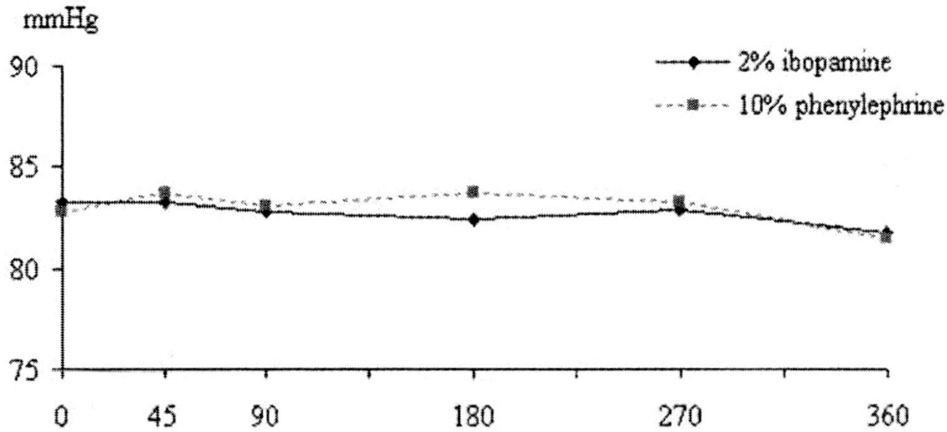

Figure 5. Glaucomatous patients - Diastolic blood pressure.

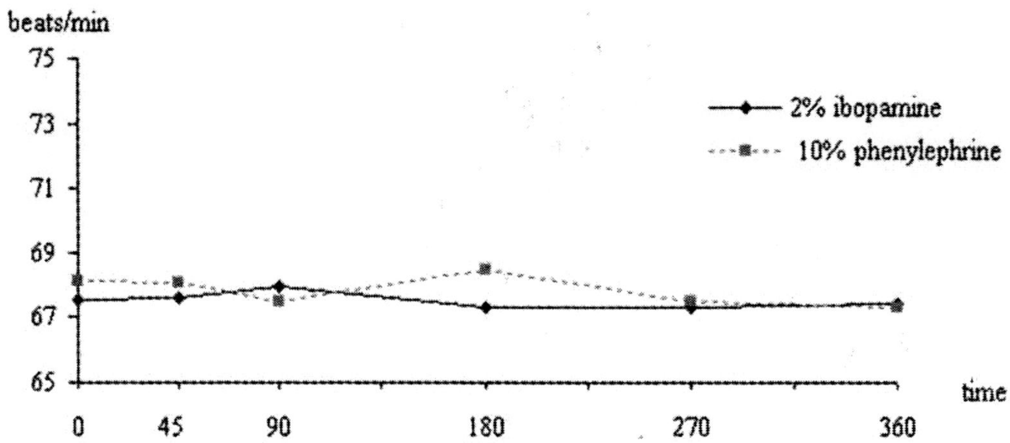

Figure 6. Glaucomatous patients - Heart rate.

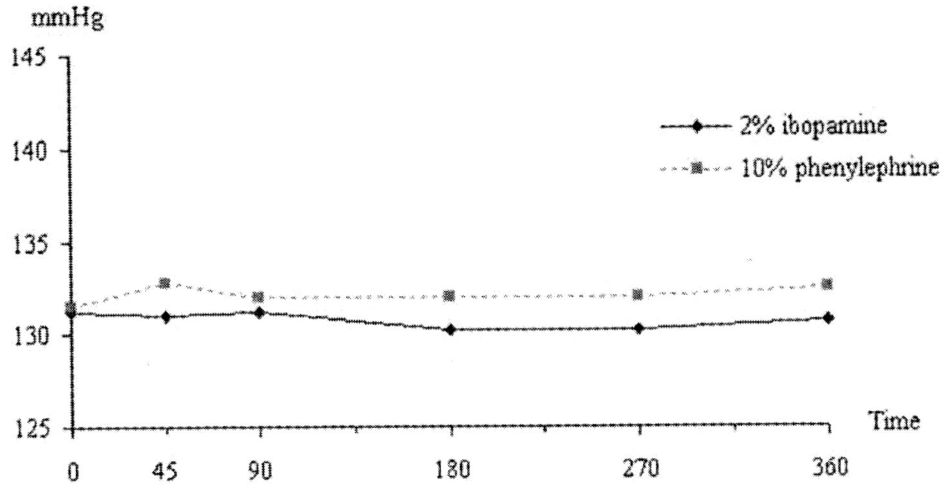

Figure 7. Healthy volunteers - Systolic blood pressure.

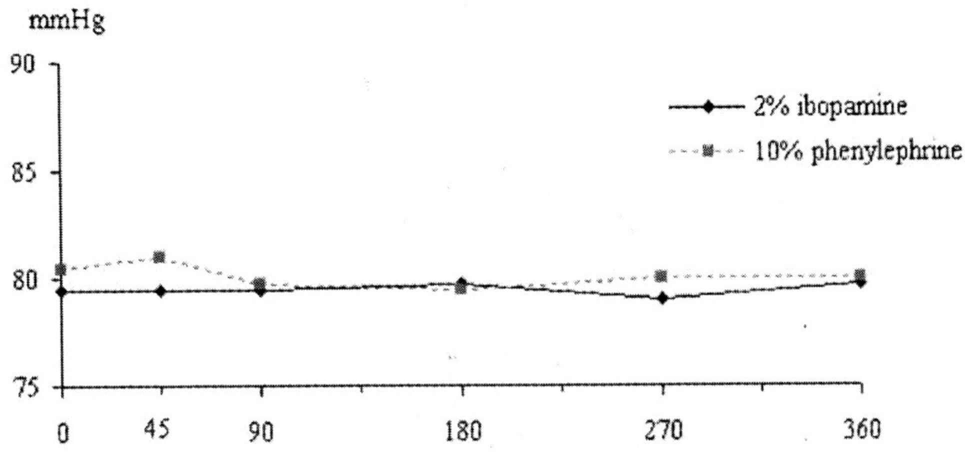

Figure 8. Healthy volunteers - Diastolic blood pressure.

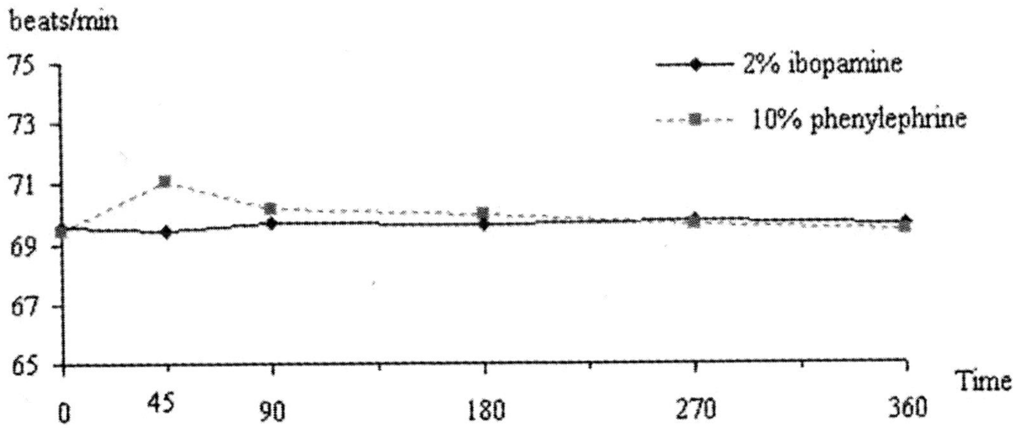

Figure 9. Healthy volunteers - Heart rate.

Receptorial Agonism

Only the D1 agonist substances, such as fenoldopam, have the same effect as ibopamine on IOP in POAG patients. D1 agonist drugs increase IOP only in POAG, but never in healthy eyes (Figure 2), assessing the involvement of D1 dopaminergic receptors on the mechanism stimulating the aqueous humor production.

Receptorial Antagonism

The hypertensive effect of ibopamine in POAG is completely counteracted by the pre-treatment with a selective antagonist of the D1 receptors: the SCH23390. A clear and definite receptorial antagonism for IOP increase has been identified. β-blockers and α-agonists [17] do not antagonize the hypertensive effects of ibopamine in POAG. Glycerol performs a partial antagonism due to an osmotic reduction of the vitreous mass.

Fluorophotometric Studies

When there is a marked increase of aqueous humor production, due to the D1 dopaminergic effect of ibopamine, the healthy eye increases its outflow thus maintaining the homeostasis; conversely in glaucomatous eyes, the impaired trabecular outflow does not maintain the hydrodynamic equilibrium and IOP increases. Fluorophotometry proves that the D1 dopaminergic stimulation, induced by 2% ibopamine, increases the aqueous humor production.

Impairment of the Outflow System in Rabbits

When inserted in the anterior chamber of the rabbit eye, Laminaria digitata induces intraocular hypertension since it impairs the outflow system. Ibopamine, when instilled, prior to the Laminaria, into the healthy rabbit eyes does not significantly affect IOP, while in the eyes treated with Laminaria digitata induces ocular hypertension.

Provocative Test in Glaucoma

Normal-tension Glaucoma

Ibopamine test resulted in IOP increase in almost 50% of cases with normal-tension glaucoma and may differentiate between eyes with normal trabecular outflow capacity and eyes with increased resistance in the trabecular meshwork that are prone to pressure peaks and deterioration to glaucoma [18].

Corticosteroid-induced Glaucoma

Long-term treatment with corticosteroids can induce ocular hypertension. They increase IOP by interfering with the aqueous humor outflow system. By administering dexamethasone at two different concentrations (0,1 and 1%) in eyes suffering from allergic conjunctivitis, the ibopamine test was positive, in a dose-dependent manner, from 33 to 50% [19].

Ibopamine in Pseudoexfoliative Syndrome

Ibopamine is useful even in detecting an impairment of the outflow system in patients affected by pseudoexfoliative syndrome (PEX) [20]. This test is positive also when PEX syndrome is unilateral.

Ibopamine Test in Children of One Glaucomatous Parent

A high percentage of positivity (about 30%) to the ibopamine test was obtained in eyes of children of one glaucomatous parent, even teenager. It is possible that these ibopamine test positive subjects, because of outflow impairment, are likely to show a clinically significant ocular hypertension or glaucoma in some years [21].

Treatment of Ocular Hypotony

Ocular hypotony is a pathological condition of the IOP homeostatic mechanisms: IOP decreases to values below 6-7 mmHg. IOP values below 4 mmHg usually cause progressive damage to the eye [22,23]. Ocular hypotony can be caused by a damage to the ciliary body from trauma, uveitis or vitreoretinal surgery [6]. Fluorophotometric studies show that 2% ibopamine induces an increase of the aqueous humor flow and production. Ibopamine can induce higher success rates in filtering surgery. In the treatment of ocular hypotony ibopamine can be administered twice daily increasing the IOP for a period of over 8 hours, associated to corticosteroids therapy.

Conclusion

In conclusion, we can consider 2% ibopamine eye drops as a useful pharmacological tool allowing us to study the pathophysiology of hydrodynamic disorders and in evaluating the outflow impairment. It is useful as a therapeutic drug in ocular hypotony secondary to filtering surgery, vitreo-retinal surgery, long-lasting uveitis and penetrating trauma.

References

[1] Virno M, Taverniti L, Motolese E et al. Ibopamina: nuovo midriatico non cicloplegico (nota preliminare). *Boll Ocul* 1986; 65: 11-2.

[2] Virno M, Pecori-Giraldi J, Taverniti L, De Gregorio F, Sedran L. Ibopamine. *D1-dopaminergic agonist in the physiopathology of intraocular pressure.* Publisher Innovation-News-Communication (I.N.C.), Rome 2003.

[3] Giuffre' I. Ibopamine stimulates α-adrenergic receptors and D1 dopaminergic receptors in the eye. *Current Drug Therapy* 2007, 2 (2): 1-6.

[4] Magacho L, Costa ML, Dessimoni A, de Avila MP. Comparison between the 1% and 2% ibopamine provocative test in primary open-angle glaucoma patients: sensitivity, specificity and tolerability. *Arq Bras Oftalmol* 2006; 69 (5): 695-9.

[5] Soldati L, Gianesello V, Galbiati I, Gazzaniga A, Virno M. Ocular pharmacokinetics and pharmacodynamics in rabbits of ibopamine, a new midriatic agent. *Exp Eye Res* 1993; 56: 247-54.

[6] Ugahary LC, Ganteris E, Veckeneer M et al. Topical ibopamine in the treatment of chronic ocular hypotony attributable to vitreoretinal surgery, uveitis, or penetrating trauma. *Am J Ophthalmol* 2006; 141: 571-3.

[7] Virno M, De Gregorio F, Grechi G et al. Azione dell'ibopamina sulla dinamica dell'umore acqueo: indagine fluorofotometrica. *Boll Ocul* 1992; 71 (suppl. 2): 103-10.

[8] Taverniti L, Di Staso S, Arrico L, D'Ubaldo E, Grenga R. The ibopamine test in patients affected by monolateral pseudoexfoliative glaucoma. *Acta Ophthalmol Scandinavica* 2000; 78: 9-11.

[9] De Gregorio F, Saccucci S, D'Ubaldo E, Virno M. Effect of repeated administration of ibopamine (D1 agonist) on IOP. *ARVO Abstract,* 1997.

[10] Azevedo H, Ciarniello MG, Rosignoli MT et al. Effects of ibopamine eye drops on intraocular pressure and aqueous humour flow in healthy volunteers and patients with open-angle glaucoma. *Eur J Ophthalmol,* 2003; 13: 370-6.

[11] Brubaker RF, McLaren J, Herman D et al. Effect of ibopamine on aqueous humour flow in normal human eyes. *Abstract ARVO,* 2003, May 4-9, Ft. Lauderdale, Florida.

[12] Giuffre' I, Taverniti L, Di Staso S. The effects of 2% ibopamine eye drops on the intraocular pressure and pupil motility of patients with open-angle glaucoma. *Eur J Ophthalmol* 2004; 14; 6: 508-13.

[13] Marchini G, Babighian S, Tosi R et al. Comparative study of the effects of 2% ibopamine, 10% phenylephrine, and 1% tropicamide on the anterior segment. *Invest Ophthalmol Vis Sci* 2003; 44: 281-9.

[14] Boles Carenini B, Brogliatti B, Boles Carenini A et al. Ibopamine: a new drug and its use as provocative test for the diagnosis of glaucoma. *New Trends in Ophthalmology* 1992; 7: 3.

[15] Nuti A, Ciappetta R, Diadori A, Frezzotti R. Ibopamine provocative test in the diagnosis of hydrodynamic disorders. *Exp Eye Res* 1992; 55 (suppl): S185.

[16] Magacho L, Costa ML, Reis R, Rios N, de Avila MP. Correlation between the ibopamine provocative test and the diurnal tension curve in glaucoma patients. *Arq Bras Oftalmol* 2006; 69 (4): 477-80.

[17] Virno M, Pecori-Giraldi J, Taverniti L et al. Indagini sul meccanismo d'azione dell'aumento tensionale di ibopamina nell'iperteso oculare. *Boll Ocul* 1989; 68 (suppl. 2): 379-84.

[18] Kniestedt C, Romppainen T, Gloor BP, Sturmer J. Positive ibopamine provocative test in normal-tension glaucoma suspects. *Klin Monatsbl Augenheilkd* 2007; 224 (4): 255-9.

[19] De Gregorio F, Arrico L, Pannarale L, Virno M. Ocular hydrodynamic disorder induced by topical steroids revealed by means of ibopamine. *ARVO Abstract,* 1995.

[20] Di Staso S, D'Andrea D, Giuffre' I et al. Test dell'ibopamina nella sindrome da pseudoesfoliazione. *Boll Ocul* 1994; 73 (suppl. 2): 325-30.

[21] Pecori Giraldi J, Damiano A, Gabrielli A et al. Ocular hypertension induced by ibopamine early discloses glaucoma suspects among relatives of glaucomatous patients. *Boll Ocul* 2002; 81: 91-5.

[22] Pannarale L, Arrico L, De Gregorio F et al. Ipotonia oculare: prospettive farmacologiche. *Boll Ocul* 1995; 74 (suppl. 2): 335-44.

[23] Pivetti Pezzi P, Da Dalt S, La Cava M, Pinca M, De Gregorio F, Virno M. Ibopamine treatment in chronic hypotony secondary to long-lasting uveitis. A case report. *Eur J Ophthalmol* 2000; 10: 332-4.

In: Research Progress on Epinephrine
Editors: A. G. Lawson and R. I. Gorman, pp. 25-41
ISBN: 978-1-60456-443-3

Chapter I

Intact Environmental Habituation and Epinephrine-Induced Enhancement of Memory Consolidation for a Novel Object Recognition Task in Pre-Weanling Sprague-Dawley Rats

Robert W. Flint, Jr., Shelby Hickey, and Maryann Dobrowolski
The College of Saint Rose, Albany, NY 12203-1490, USA

Abstract

Within- and between-session environmental habituation were examined in infant rats on postnatal days 14 and 15 in an open field. Using a computerized animal tracking system, rats showed decreases in the total distance traveled (m) and overall average speed (m/s) across 6 30-sec time blocks each day and from day 1 to day 2 of testing. Although the literature is inconclusive regarding the ontogeny of environmental habituation, these results provide clear evidence of both within-session and between-session habituation. On postnatal day 16, animals were returned to the open field with 2 identical objects for novel object recognition training. Animals were either tested immediately after training or were given a subcutaneous injection of saline or .01 mg/kg of epinephrine, followed by testing 2-hrs later. For testing, animals were placed into the open field with one familiar and one novel object, and the number of object explorations and the time spent exploring each object were recorded by the animal tracking system. From these measures the absolute mean preference for novelty and relative percent preference for novelty were computed. Only the relative percent preference for novelty based on the time spent exploring each object revealed significant differences among the groups. Post-hoc pair-wise comparisons indicated that saline animals tested 2-hrs after training performed significantly worse than epinephrine animals and worse than those tested immediately after training. This indicates a rapid rate of forgetting for object recognition memory which is effectively attenuated with post-training epinephrine.

Introduction

Age-related memory impairments are stereotypically thought of as afflicting the elderly, and are infrequently a concern for children, young adults, or even those of middle-age. However, we have all suffered and continue to suffer from a very significant form of memory loss described by Freud (1914/1938) as infantile amnesia. Research examining the ontogeny of memory encompasses some very important endeavors in behavioral and developmental neuroscience. The goal of the present study was to examine environmental habituation and object recognition memory in preweanling rats and to determine the effect of epinephrine on novel object recognition memory.

Immature mammals commonly exhibit a rapid rate of forgetting (Arnold & Spear, 1997; Campbell & Campbell, 1962; Campbell, Jaynes, & Misanin, 1968; Campbell & Spear, 1972; Hartshorn et al., 1998; Kirby, 1963; Spear & Riccio, 1994; Spear & Rudy, 1991) and an inability to accurately recall events from infancy after reaching adulthood (Freud, 1914/1938; Sheingold & Tenney, 1982; Usher & Neisser, 1993; see Pillemer & White, 1989 for review). While both of these phenomena may be described as infantile amnesia, the present study was interested in the characteristics of the former mnemonic deficit, namely that immature organisms rapidly forget recently learned information. For example, Hill, Borovsky, and Rovee-Collier (1988) used 6-7-month-old human infants and demonstrated that they could acquire and maintain a memory for an operant conditioning procedure for 14 days, but that complete forgetting of the procedure would occur by 21 days post-training.

It is paradoxical that this critical period of development is associated with such poor memory. The cause of infantile amnesia is not known, but Campbell and Spear (1972) and Howe and Courage (1993) reviewed a variety of potential mechanisms for this phenomenon. In humans it was suggested that the development of a cognitive sense of self, along with the personalization of event memory are particularly important. Other proposed mechanisms that are not limited to humans included maturational changes in interference and information-processing and neuroanatomical and/or biochemical changes in the central nervous system. While the cause of infantile amnesia continues to be debated, increased knowledge of biological ontogentic changes makes this a plausible consideration. For example, it is well-known that both the limbic system, a group of interconnected neuroanatomical structures heavily involved in learning and memory, and the hypothalamic-pituitary-adrenal axis are developmentally immature (Bayer & Altman, 1975; Levine, 1994; Schapiro, Geller, & Eiduson, 1962; Schlessinger, Cowan, & Gottlieb, 1975; Schmidt et al., 2003; Vazquez, 1998).

Regardless of the cause of this rapid rate of forgetting, research has clearly indicated that this deficit is the result of a retrieval failure at the time of testing, and not a failure to learn the material during training. This is evidenced by the success of treatments to enhance the retrieval of memories formed during infancy (Anderson, Karash, & Riccio, 2001; Campbell & Jaynes, 1966; Flint, Bunsey, & Riccio, 1999; Flint & Riccio, 1997; Greco, Rovee-Collier, Hayne, Griesler, & Earley, 1986; Hamberg, & Spear, 1978; Rovee-Collier & Hayne, 1987; Rovee-Collier, Sullivan, Enright, Lucas, & Fagan, 1980; Richardson, Wang, & Campbell, 1993). Spear and Parsons (1976) trained rats at postnatal day 16, postnatal day 23, or as adults and tested them 28 days later. They demonstrated that an unconditioned stimulus

(UCS; footshock) reactivation treatment 24-hours prior to testing had differential effects on retention performance based on the age at which training occurred. The reactivation treatment was effective for all groups with the exception of the 16-day-old animals. However, Spear and Parsons did find that the reactivation treatment was effective for subjects at this age if the retention interval was shortened to 7 days instead of 28 days. These results indicate that the training memory was stored, but the effectiveness of the reactivation treatment likely decreases as the retention interval increases. Furthermore, a single exposure to the conditioning reinforcer was sufficient to reactivate the training memory.

The creation and use of new memories involves a complex series of processes including information acquisition, consolidation, storage, and retrieval, with distinct biochemical processes and neuroanatomical substrates which may differ depending upon the nature of the to-be-remembered information. Research indicates that memory consolidation is a time-limited event occurring immediately following acquisition. During this time the memory is in a labile state where manipulations may either enhance or impair the consolidation process, resulting in either enhanced or impaired performance on subsequent tests. For example, some memory enhancing treatments in rats include adrenocorticotropic hormone (Gold & van Buskirk, 1976), glucose (Flint & Riccio, 1996; 1999; Gold, 1986), vasopressin (Koob et al., 1991), oxytocin (Bohus, Conti, Kovacs, & Versteeg, 1982), gastrointestinal peptides (Morley & Flood, 1991), and epinephrine (Costa-Miserachs, Portell-Cortes, Aldavert-Vera, Torras-Garcia, & Morgado-Bernal, 1994; Gold & van Buskirk, 1975, 1978; Nordby, Torras-Garcia, Portel-Cortes, & Costa-Miserachs, 2006). Of paramount importance to the present study are those experiments demonstrating the memory enhancing effects of epinephrine when administered immediately following training.

Post-training epinephrine has been shown to enhance memory consolidation for a variety of tasks including inhibitory avoidance conditioning (Gold & van Buskirk, 1975, 1978), taste conditioning (Guaza, Borrell, & Borrell, 1986), appetitive conditioning (Sternberg, Isaacs, Gold, & McGaugh, 1985), and novel object recognition memory (Dornelles et al., 2007). Gold, Murphy, and Cooley (1982) trained 16-day-old rats on an inhibitory avoidance conditioning task. They found that these animals demonstrated good retention of the training shortly afterwards (1-hr) but not 24-hrs later, evidence of infantile amnesia. A subcutaneous injection of epinephrine immediately after training enhanced subsequent performance on the retention test 24-hrs later. In a more recent study, Flint, Bunsey, and Riccio (2007) examined the effects of epinephrine on memory retrieval of inhibitory avoidance conditioning in 17-day-old rats. Animals that had received a subcutaneous injection of .01 mg/kg or .1 mg/kg of epinephrine 25 ($\pm$5-min) prior to the retention test exhibited significantly better retention scores. Importantly, control groups indicated that these results were not likely due to the effects of epinephrine on vigilance or as an internal contextual reminder cue of training.

In novel object recognition memory, animals are commonly presented with two identical objects in an open field type apparatus. Animals are given a specific amount of time to freely explore these objects. On a subsequent retention test, animals are presented with two objects, one familiar (from training) and one novel, and are similarly free to explore these objects. Animals with intact object recognition memory will spend more time exploring the novel object, indicating intact retention of the familiar object (Anderson et al., 2004; Ennaceur & Delacour, 1988; Steckler, Drinkenburg, Sahgal, & Aggleton, 1998). Dornelles et al. (2007)

utilized the object recognition paradigm with adult rats. Animals exposed to the training objects for 2-min showed intact memory during the recognition test 1.5 or 24 hours later, but not 96 hours following training. Immediate post-training administration of epinephrine attenuated this recognition memory deficit when tested 96 hours after training.

Unlike environmental habituation, object recognition memory requires the animal to establish a memory for a specific environmental stimulus. Since it is common to provide animals with a chance to acclimate to the apparatus prior to training in tasks like novel object recognition (Besheer & Bevins, 2000), the present study took advantage of this opportunity to examine environmental habituation on postnatal days 14 and 15. Prior reports examining the ontogeny of environmental habituation have provided in inconsistent results. Ba and Seri (1995) examined head-dip responses on a hole-board test in animals between postnatal day 10 and 45. They did not find any evidence of within-session habituation at postnatal days 10 or 15, but environmental habituation was evident at 20-days-of-age. Similar results have also been reported by Feigley, Parsons, Hamilton, and Spear (1972). In contrast, File (1978) used the head-dip response to examine the ontogeny of habituation and found that 16-day-old animals demonstrated both within- and between-session environmental habituation. Using an open field apparatus, Bronstein, Neiman, Wolkoff, and Levine (1974) recorded the number of grid crossings and the duration of horizontal movement in 15-, 21-, and 100-day-old rats. They found that 21- and 100-day-old animals habituated to the open field, but there was no evidence of within-session habituation in 15-day-old animals.

In the present study we examined the locomotor activity of 14- and 15-day-old animals in an open field for evidence of within- and between-session environmental habituation. On postnatal day 16, animals were returned to the open field for novel object recognition training. Animals were either tested for novel object recognition memory immediately after training, or were given a subcutaneous injection of saline or epinephrine followed by testing 2 hours later. No hypotheses were formulated regarding environmental habituation, given the lack of consensus in the literature. Based upon evidence indicating that epinephrine effectively attenuates infantile amnesia for avoidance conditioning and enhances object recognition memory in adult rats, we hypothesized that immediate posttraining injection of epinephrine would enhance subsequent retention performance.

Methods

Subjects

Fifty-nine (37 male, 22 female) Sprague-Dawley rat pups from 5 litters were used for this study. Animals were bred from Harlan Lab breeding stock at The College of Saint Rose. Litters were culled at 5-6 days-of-age to 11-12 pups per litter and were maintained in large Plexiglas cages with dam, food, and water for the duration of the study. The colony room was kept at approximately 70° F on a reversed 9:15 hr light:dark cycle. All testing took place during the dark phase of the cycle. The date of birth was counted as day 0 when determining the age of the animals. Animals were handled for 3-min each on postnatal days 12 and 13 and all animals had their eyes open on day 14. Animals were weighed at postnatal day 16

(M=30.90 g, SE=.45 g) shortly prior to injection to ensure that injection volumes were accurate. All experimental procedures were approved by the Institutional Animal Care and Use Committee prior to the onset of the study.

Materials and Apparatus

The open field apparatus consisted of a round aluminum tub, within which a 54.0 cm diameter 2.0 cm thick board was inserted. Both the board and the aluminum tub were painted with multiple coats of black paint to seal the surfaces as well as provide a background on which animals would be easily visible. The walls of the apparatus were 25.4 cm high and the room was illuminated with overhead fluorescent lighting. A 68 dB white noise was present during all exposures to the apparatus to mask background noises. A total of four objects were used for training and testing on the novel object recognition task (2 identical green plastic bolts and 2 identical purple plastic Mega Bloks^{TM}). The green plastic bolt (circular base diameter = 3.5 cm, height = 6.4 cm) and a purple plastic Mega Blok^{TM} (square base width = 3.2, height = 3.5) were selected from a set of objects based on pilot data that indicated equivalent preferences for the two objects. Objects were mounted onto small pieces of black Plexiglas (5.1 x 7.6 cm) with bolts extending from the bottom, that allowed them to be fitted into small pre-drilled holes on the base of the open field. Objects were positioned in the middle of the apparatus 20.3 cm apart on center. The apparatus and objects were thoroughly cleaned with disinfectant after each animal in order to eliminate the potential effect of scent marks left by prior animals.

Pre-training habituation sessions, training, and testing were recorded using the AnyMaze animal tracking system (Stoelting, Inc., Wood Dale, IL). The AnyMaze software was loaded onto a standard IBM office computer to which a digital camera was attached and suspended directly above the open field apparatus. Using the AnyMaze system, the open field was divided into 3 zones, the first zone contained the entire visible area of the open field (2289 cm^2), the second zone measured 10.2 cm by 12.7 cm and encompassed the first object, and the third zone with the same dimensions encompassed the second object. The total distance traveled (m), overall average speed (m/s), number of entries into the object zones, and the time spent in the object zones (s) were recorded as dependent measures. Silvers, Harrod, Ferris, Mactutus, and Booze (2006) have demonstrated that the use of automated animal tracking systems produces the same pattern of results for object novelty tasks as coding dependent upon experimenter observation.

Sterile saline (.85% NaCl) or epinephrine (.01 mg/kg; Sigma Chemical Co., St. Louis, MO) were administered subcutaneously in the nape of the neck at a volume of 1 ml/kg. The dose of epinephrine was selected based on extensive literature indicating that this concentration is optimal for enhancing memory consolidation (Costa-Miserachs, Portell-Cortes, Aldavert-Vera, Torras-Garcia, & Morgado-Bernal, 1994; Flint, Bunsey, & Riccio, 2007; Nordby, Torras-Garcia, Portell-Cortes, & Costa-Miserachs, 2006; Williams, Men, Clayton, & Gold, 1998).

Procedure

Animals were handled for 3-min each on postnatal days 12 and 13 in order to acclimate them to being handled. On postnatal days 14 and 15, animals were placed individually into the open field apparatus without any objects present. Animals remained in the apparatus for 3-min during which AnyMaze tracked their behavior. This 2-day pre-training phase was used to acclimate the animals to the apparatus and to specifically examine these animals for within- and between-session environmental habituation. For all pre-training, training, and testing sessions animals were placed onto the center of the open field at the beginning of the session.

On postnatal day 16, animals were pseudorandomly assigned to one of 3 groups, so that 3-4 animals from each litter were represented in each group. Animals in the immediate test group (n=16) were tested immediately after training. Animals in the saline group (n=12) and the epinephrine group (n=17) were administered their respective subcutaneous injection immediately after training, followed by a 2-hr delay before testing was conducted. Training for all animals involved being placed into the center of the open field for 3-min in the presence of 2 identical objects. Designation of the training objects (green bolts or purple Mega Bloks^{TM}) was randomly counterbalanced across subjects. Testing for all animals involved being returned to the apparatus with one familiar object (from training) and one novel object (never seen before) for 3-min. The placement of the familiar and novel objects (left/right) was counterbalanced across animals. AnyMaze recorded the behavior of the animals during all phases of the study.

Results

Results were analyzed using parametric tests and were considered significant when *p* was less than or equal to .05. Partial eta squared (η_p^2) has been reported as an effect-size statistic for all omnibus analysis of variance (ANOVA) tests and Cohen's d (*d*; Faul, Erdfelder, Lang, & Buchner, 2007) has been reported for pairwise analyses. Post-hoc power analyses have also been tabulated for all results that failed to reach statistical significance.

Pretraining Locomotor Activity

All animals were given 3-min sessions to explore the apparatus once at 14-days-old and again at 15-days-old during which the distance traveled and overall average speed were determined (see Figures 1 and 2). Each session was divided into 6 30-sec time blocks (epochs). A 2x2x6 (sex x day x epoch) mixed ANOVA for total distance traveled (m) revealed a significant effect of day [$F(1,57)=38.26$, $p<.001$, $\eta_p^2=.40$], a significant effect of epoch [Huynh-Feldt Correction $F(4.44,252.91)=45.27$, $p<.001$, $\eta_p^2=.44$], and a significant day by epoch interaction [Huynh-Feldt Correction $F(4.76,271.10)=3.84$, $p<.01$, $\eta_p^2=.06$]. There was no main effect of sex [$F(1,57)=1.25$, $p>.05$, $\eta_p^2=.02$, power=.20]. Analyses of the overall average speed (m/s) revealed the same pattern of results. A 2x2x6 (sex x day x epoch) mixed ANOVA for total distance traveled indicated a main effect of day [$F(1,57)=38.90$, $p<.001$, $\eta_p^2=.41$], a main effect of epoch [Huynh-Feldt Correction $F(4.42,251.70)=45.38$, $p<.001$, $\eta_p^2=.44$], and a significant day by epoch interaction [Huynh-Feldt Correction $F(4.74,270.13)=4.12$, $p=.002$, $\eta_p^2=.07$]. There was no main effect of sex [$F(1,57)=1.26$, $p>.05$, $\eta_p^2=.02$, power=.20].

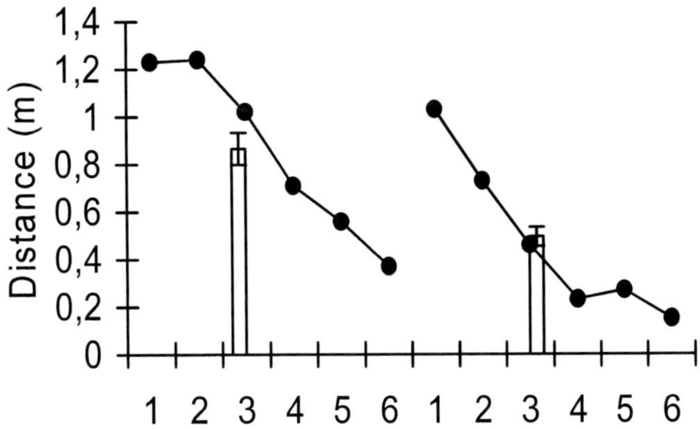

Figure 1. Lines represent the mean total distance traveled (m) during each of the 6 30-sec epochs at 14- and 15-days-of-age. Bars represent the mean total distance traveled on each day. Error bars represent the standard error of the mean.

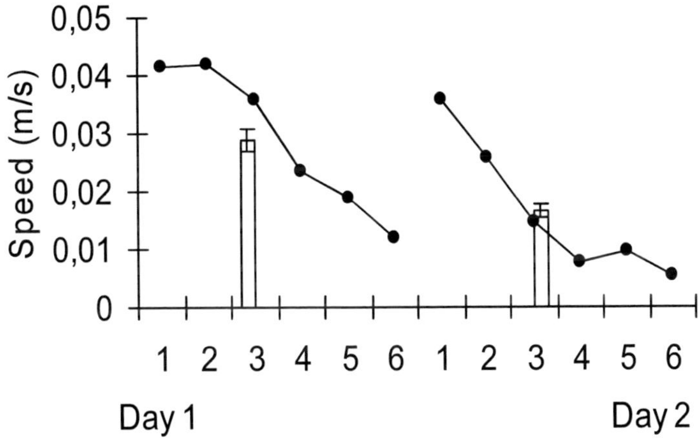

Figure 2. Lines represent the mean overall average speed (m/s) during each of the 6 30-sec epochs at 14- and 15-days-of-age. Bars represent the mean overall average speed on each day. Error bars represent the standard error of the mean.

Object Recognition

The absolute mean preference for novelty (novel minus familiar) and the relative percent preference for novelty [(novel/total) x 100] for the immediate test, saline control, and epinephrine groups were calculated for both the number of object zone entries and the time spent exploring each object. A 2x3 (sex x group) ANOVA on the absolute mean preference for novelty did not reveal any significant effects using the number of explorations [Sex $F(1,39)=1.40$, $p>.05$, power=.21; Group $F(2,39)=1.31$, $p>.05$, power=.27] or the time spent exploring [Sex $F(1,39)=.01$, $p>.05$, power=.05; Group $F(2,39)=1.51$, $p>.05$, power=.30]. ANOVAs for the relative percent preference for novelty, similarly, did not reveal any significant effects using the number of explorations [Sex $F(1,39)=.24$, $p>.05$, power=.08; Group $F(2,39)=1.44$, $p>.05$, power=.29]. However, a significant effect of group for the relative percent preference for novelty on time spent object exploring was revealed [$F(2,39)=5.00$, $p<.05$, $\eta_p^2=.20$] (see Figure 3). Post-hoc Fischer's LSD tests for pairwise comparisons revealed that the saline control tested 2-hrs after training had a significantly lower percent preference score in comparison to both the immediate test group and the epinephrine group tested 2-hrs after training. There was no significant effect of sex for the relative percent preference score [$F(1,39)=.52$, $p>.05$, power=.11].

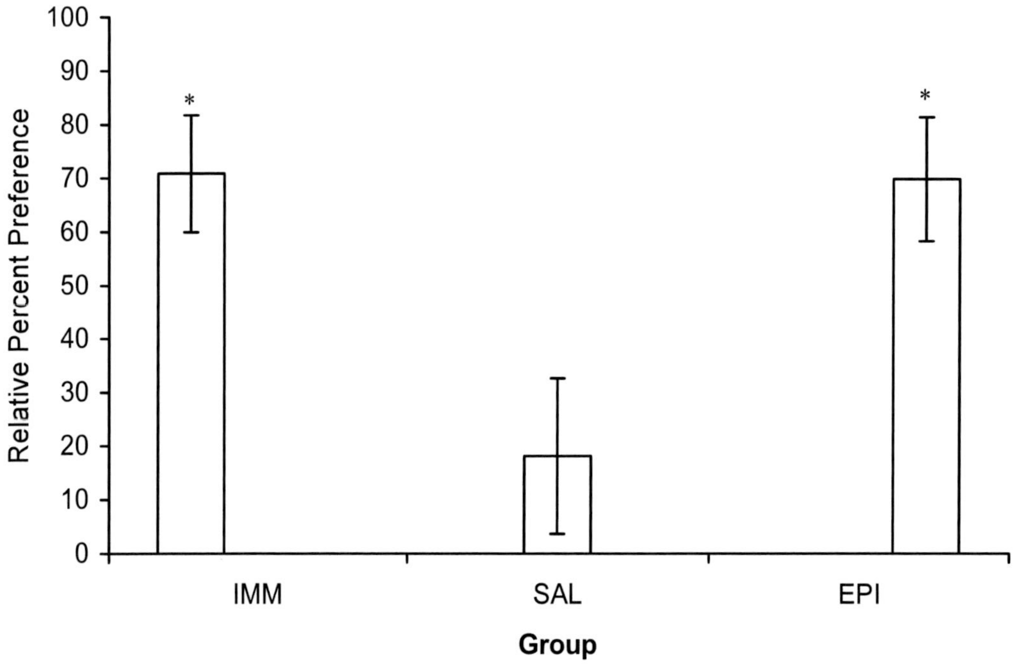

Figure 3. Mean relative percent preference for object exploration time for the immediate test, saline, and epinephrine groups. Error bars represent the standard error of the mean.

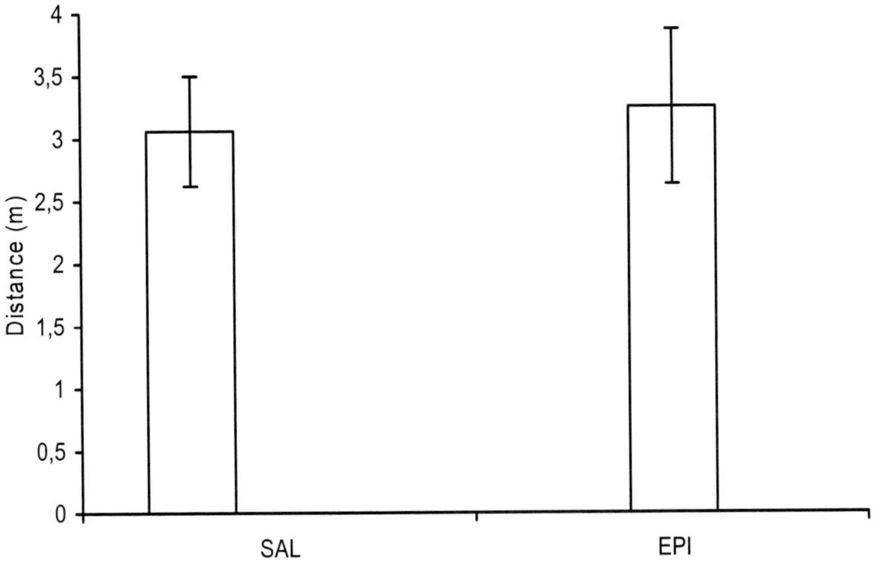

Figure 4. Mean total distance traveled (m) for the saline and epinephrine groups during the novel object recognition test on postnatal day 16. Error bars represent the standard error of the mean.

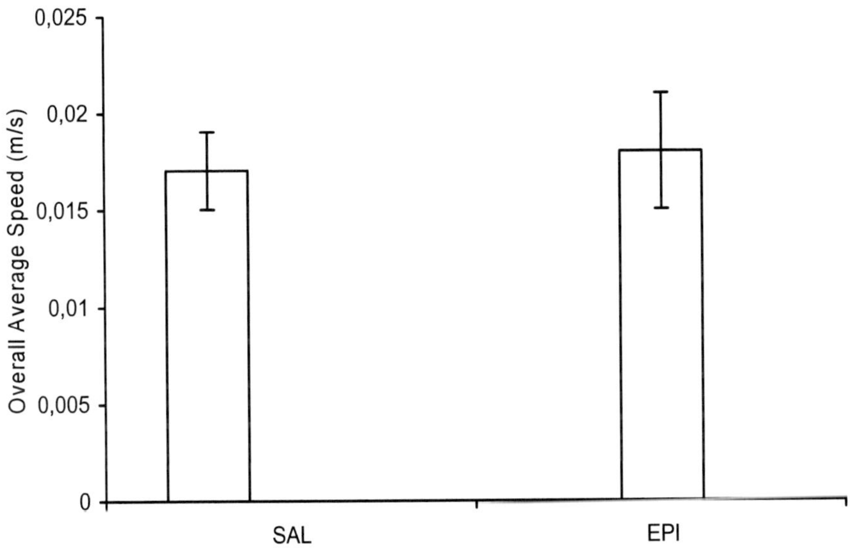

Figure 5. Mean overall average speed (m/s) for the saline and epinephrine groups during the novel object recognition test on postnatal day 16. Error bars represent the standard error of the mean.

Locomotor Activity during Testing

Since testing was conducted two hours following training in the saline and epinephrine groups, it is possible that residual effects of epinephrine might have elevated activity levels confounding the results. In order to examine this potential confound, the test data for male and female animals were combined, as prior analyses did not reveal any sex differences.

Independent samples t-tests for the total distance traveled [$t(38)=.25$, $p>.05$, $d=.45$, power=.28] and overall average speed [$t(38)=.23$, $p>.05$, $d=.00001$, power=.05] did not reveal any differences between the saline and the epinephrine groups (see Figures 4 and 5).

Conclusions

Early studies of environmental habituation depended upon manual coding, frequently involving counting the number of times animals crossed lines on the grid floor of an apparatus. With the advent of computerized animal tracking systems we are now able to obtain detailed measurements such as the exact distance traveled and the average speed providing a more accurate measure of exploratory behavior and activity level. In the present study, open field activity measures in animals at postnatal days 14 and 15 showed significant within- and between-session environmental habituation. The total distance traveled and the overall average speed declined across the 6 30-sec epochs within the test sessions on each day, and there was a significant reduction in these measures from day 1 to day 2. These changes in behavior indicate that at postnatal day 14, animals are capable of forming a memory of their environment and maintaining it for at least 24-hrs. Similar within- and between-session habituation results have been reported using head-dipping as a dependent measure in 16-day-old rats (File, 1978) and Goodwin and Barr (1997) have reported envorinmental habituation of locmotor activity at postnatal day 10. However, our results are in contrast to those reported by Bronstein, Neiman, Wolkoff, and Levine (1974) in a study of the ontogeny of environmental habituation (see also Feigley, Parsons, Hamilton, & Spear, 1972). The reason for this difference is not clear, but our study differs on many levels including the method of data collection, the size of the groups, and behavioral protocol.

Based, in part, upon earlier studies failing to show sufficient environmental habituation in immature animals, some researchers have suggested that this apparent behavioral deficit may be a result of an immature hippocampal system (Bronstein et al., 1974) or underdeveloped cholinergic inhibitory mechanism (Feigley et al., 1972). Carman and Mactutus (2001) used the water maze to investigate the ontogeny of spatial navigation in rats. A critical manipulation they made was to adjust the size of the apparatus to that of the developmental size of the animal. Using this technique, they were able to demonstrate that 17-day-old preweanling animals show evidence of learning in a water maze 1/3 the size of that used for adults. Based upon these data, Carman and Mactutus suggested that the developmentally immature state of the hippocampus in 17-day-old preweanling rats did not preclude its ability to integrate visual-spatial information. This hypothesis is important to the present study, as environmental habituation and novel object recognition memory are hippocampal-dependent tasks. If Carman and Mactutus are correct, it is logical to expect that the developmental state of the hippocampus between 14 and 16 days may similarly be sufficient to allow for visual-spatial learning. More importantly, it appears as though environmental habituation may be retained for at least 24-hours, similar to those reported by Carman and Mactutus using the water maze.

Results of the object recognition memory task indicate that epinephrine administered immediately following training attenuated the memory deficit seen in these infant animals according to relative percent preference scores for the time spent exploring the objects. It is important to note that overall average speed and distance traveled during the object recognition memory test did not differ between groups, suggesting that there were no residual effects of epinephrine present. Additional support for this comes from the finding that absolute novelty preference scores, known to be sensitive to differences in activity levels, did not reflect any group differences. Epinephrine has a very short half-life and reaches peak plasma levels following stress in less than 1 minute (Berne & Levy, 1993; Dimsdale & Moss, 1980; Steptoe, 1987) in humans, so if plasma levels are similar in rats it is unlikely that epinephrine would have influenced locomotor activity 2-hrs following administration.

Although considerable evidence indicates that epinephrine enhances memory consolidation (Introini-Collison & McGaugh, 1991; McGaugh, 1983; McGaugh & Roozendaal, 2002), two studies by Izquierdo and colleagues have suggested that epinephrine may sometimes prevent the disruptive effects of retroactive interference (Izquierdo, Barcik, & Brioni, 1989; Izquierdo & Pereira, 1989). In their studies, the disruptive effects of post-training (conditioned emotional responding or inhibitory avoidance conditioning) exposure to an open field or extinction session were prevented with epinephrine administration. However, Izquierdo and Pereira did report that the retroactive interference produced by a series of tones presented following inhibitory avoidance conditioning was not attenuated by post-training epinephrine administration. It is therefore possible that post-training epinephrine effects on subsequent memory performance may, in part, be due to increased resistance to retroactive interference.

One potential mechanism of epinephrine-induced memory modulation involves the subsequent elevation in blood glucose level. Epinephrine does not easily cross the blood brain barrier (Axelrod, Weil-Malherbe, & Tomchick, 1959), but glucose does. Epinephrine affects the liver which in turn may then affect the pancreas, both leading to an elevation in blood glucose level (Flint, 2002). It is not clear whether or not this potential mechanism is intact and functional in 16-day-old rats. The development of the pancreas is ongoing following birth (Bourassa et al, 1999; Hill, Hogg, Petrik, Arany, & Han, 1999; Lu, Lebenthal, & Lee, 1987) and these immature animals are primarily utilizing ketones for energy at this age as opposed to glucose (Vannucci & Simpson, 2003). The later developmental switch from ketones to glucose is accompanied by elevations in glucose transporters in the brain (Vannucci, 1994; Vannucci et al., 1998; Vannucci, Seaman, Brucklacher, & Vannucci, 1994; Vannucci, Willing, & Vannucci, 1993) which recent evidence suggests may be important for memory (Choeiri, Staines, Miki, Seino, and Messier, 2005). Other mechanisms of epinephrine-induced memory modulation may include indirect effects on the nucleus tractus solitarius, basolateral nucleus of the amygdala, locus coeruleus, and the hippocampus (Clayton & Williams, 2000ab; Ferry, Roozendaal, & McGaugh, 1993; Liang, McGaugh, & Yao, 1990; Miyashita & Williams, 2004; Williams & McGaugh, 1993; Williams, Men, & Clayton, 2000). Future research may help to elucidate the mechanisms of epinephrine-induced memory modulation.

References

Anderson, M. J., Barnes, G. W., Briggs, J. F., Ashton, K. M., Moody, E. W., Joynes, R. L., & Riccio, D. C. (2004). The effects of ontogeny on the performance of rats in a novel object recognition task. *Psychological Reports, 94,* 437-443.

Anderson, M. J., Karash, D. L., & Riccio, D. C. (2004). The alleviation of ontogenetic forgetting in a novel object recognition task. *Journal of Behavioral and Neuroscience Research, 2*(1), 1-5.

Arnold, H. M., & Spear, N. E. (1997). Infantile amnesia: using animal models to understand forgetting. In P. J. B. Slater, J. S. Rosenblatt, C. T. Snowden, & M. Milinski (Eds.), *Advances in the study of behavior,* vol. 26 (pp. 251-284). New York, NY: Academic Press.

Axelrod, J., Weil-Malherbe, H., & Tomchick, R. (1959). The physiological disposition of 3H-epinephrine and its metabolite metanephrine. *Journal of Pharmacology and Experimental Therapeutics, 127,* 251-256.

Ba, A., & Seri, B. V. (1995). Psychomotor functions in developing rats: ontogenetic approach to structure-function relationships. *Neuroscience and Biobehavioral Reviews, 19*(3), 413-425.

Bayer, S. A., & Altman, J. (1975). The effects of X-irradiation on the postnatally-forming granule cell populations in the olfactory bulb, hippocampus, and cerebellum of the rat. *Experimental Neurology, 48,* 167-174.

Berne, R. M., & Levy, M. N. (1993). Physiology (3rd ed.). St. Louis, MO: Mosby-Year Book, Inc.

Besheer, J., & Bevins, R. A. (2000). The role of environmental familiarization in novel-object preference. *Behavioural Processes, 50,* 19-29.

Bourassa, J., Laine, J., Marie-Luise, K., Gagnon, M. C., Calvo, E., & Morisset, J. (1999). Ontogeny and species differences in the pancreatic expression and localization of the CCKA receptors. *Biochemistry, Biophysics, and Research Communication, 260,* 820-828.

Bronstein, P. M., Neiman, H., Wolkoff, F. D., & Levine, M. J. (1974). The development of habituation in the rat. *Animal Learning & Behavior, 2*(2), 92-96.

Bohus, B., Conti, L., Kovacs, G. L., & Versteeg, D. H. G. (1982). Modulation of memory processes by neuropeptides: Interaction with neurotransmitter systems. In C. Ajmone Marsan & H. Matthies (Eds.), *Neuronal plasticity and memory formation.* New York, NY: Raven Press.

Campbell, B. A., & Campbell, E. H. (1962). Retention and extinction of learned fear in infant and adult rats. *Journal of Comparative and Physiological Psychology, 55,* 1-8.

Campbell, B. A., & Jaynes, J. (1966). Reinstatement. *Psychological Review, 73,* 478-480.

Campbell, B. A., Jaynes, J. R., & Misanin, J. (1968). Retention of a light-dark discrimination in rats of different ages. *Journal of Comparative and Physiological Psychology, 66,* 467-472.

Campbell, B. A., & Spear, N. E. (1972). Ontogeny of memory. *Psychological Review, 79,* 215-236.

Choeiri, C., Staines, W., Miki, T., Seino, S., & Messier, C. (2005). Glucose transporter plasticity during memory processing. *Neuroscience, 130,* 591-600.

Clayton, E. C., & Williams, C. L. (2000a). Adrenergic activation of the nucleus tractus solitarius potentiates amygdala norepinephrine release and enhances retention performance in emotionally arousing and spatial memory tasks. *Behavioural Brain Research, 112,* 151-158.

Clayton, E. C., & Williams, C. L. (2000b). Noradrenergic receptor blockade of the NTS attenuates the mnemonic effects of epinephrine in an appetitive light-dark discrimination learning task. *Neurobiology of Learning and Memory, 74,* 135-145.

Costa-Miserachs, D., Portell-Cortex, I., Aldavert-Vera, L., Torras-Garcia, M., & Morgado-Bernal, I. (1994). Long-term memory facilitation in rats by posttraining epinephrine. *Behavioral Neuroscience, 108*(3), 469-474.

Dimsdale, J. E., & Moss, J. (1980). Short-term catecholamine response to psychological stress. *Psychosomatic Medicine, 42*(5), 493-497.

Dornelles, A., Martins de Lima, M. N., Grazziotin, M., Presti-Torres, J., Garcia, V. A., Scalco, F. S., Roesler, R., & Schroder, N. (2007). Adrenergic enhancement of consolidation of object recognition memory. *Neurobiology of Learning and Memory, 88,* 137-142.

Ennaceur, A., & Delacour, J. (1988). A new one-trial test for neurobiological studies of memory in rats 1: Behavioral data. *Behavioural Brain Research, 31*(1), 47-59.

Faul, F., Erdfelder, E., Lang, A.-G. & Buchner, A. (2007). G*Power 3: A flexible statistical power analysis program for the social, behavioral, and biomedical sciences. *Behavior Research Methods*, 39, 175-191.

Feigley, D. A., Parsons, P. J., Hamilton, L. W., & Spear, N. E. (1972). Development of habituation to novel environments in the rat. *Journal of Comparative and Physiological Psychology, 79*(3), 443-452.

Ferry, B., Roozendaal, B., & McGaugh, J. L. (1999). Role of norepinephrine in mediating stress hormone regulation of long-term memory storage: A critical involvement of the amygdala. *Biological Psychiatry, 46,* 1140-1152.

File, S. E. (1978). The ontogeny of exploration in the rat: Habituation and effects of handling. *Developmental Psychobiology, 11*(4), 321-328.

Flint, R. W., Jr. (2002). Glucose-induced memory modulation. In R. W. Flint, Jr. (Ed.), *Forget it? Sources, theories, and mechanisms of alterations in mnemonic function* (pp. 197-216). North Chelmsford, MA: Courier Custom Publishing, Inc., Erudition Books.

Flint, R. W., Jr., Bunsey, M. D., & Riccio, D. C. (1999). UCS intensity-dependent attenuation of infantile amnesia. *Psychobiology, 27*(4), 530-540.

Flint, R. W., Jr., Bunsey, M. D., & Riccio, D. C. (2007). Epinephrine-induced enhancement of memory retrieval for inhibitory avoidance conditioning in preweanling Sprague-Dawley rats. *Developmental Psychobiology, 49*, 303-311.

Flint, R. W., Jr., & Riccio, D. C. (1996). Glucose administration attenuates hypothermia-induced retrograde amnesia in rats in a time- and dose-dependent manner. *Psychobiology, 24,* 62-66.

Flint, R. W., Jr., & Riccio, D. C. (1997). Pretest administration of glucose attenuates infantile amnesia for passive avoidance conditioning in rats. *Developmental Psychobiology, 31,* 207-216.

Flint, R. W., Jr., & Riccio, D. C. (1999). Post-training glucose administration attenuates forgetting of passive-avoidance conditioning in 18-day-old rats. *Neurobiology of Learning and Memory, 72,* 62-67.

Freud, S. (1938). The writings of Sigmund Freud (A. A. Brill, Trans.), New York, NY: Random House. (Original work published 1914)

Gold, P. E. (1986). Glucose modulation of memory storage. *Behavioral & Neural Biology, 45,* 342-349.

Gold, P. E., & van Buskirk, R. B. (1975). Facilitation of time-dependent memory processes with posttrial epinephrine injections. *Behavioral Biology, 13,* 145-153.

Gold, P. E., & van Buskirk, R. B. (1976). Enhancement and impairment of memory processes with post-trial injections of adrenocorticotropic hormone. *Behavioral Biology, 16,* 387-400.

Gold, P. E., & van Buskirk, R. B. (1978). Effects of alpha- and beta-adrenergic receptor antagonists on posttrial epinephrine modulation of memory: Relationship to posttraining brain norepinephrine concentrations. *Behavioral Biology, 24,* 1168-1184.

Goodwin, G. A., & Barr, G. A. (1997). Evidence for opioid and nonopioid processes mediating adaptive responses of infant rats that are repeatedly isolated. *Developmental Psychobiology, 31,* 217-227.

Greco, C., Rovee-Collier, C., Hayne, H., Griesler, P., & Earley, L. (1986). Ontogeny of early event memory: I. Forgetting and retrieval by 2- and 3-month-olds. *Infant Behavior Development, 9,* 441-460.

Guaza, C., Borrell, S., & Borrell, J. (1986). Effects of adrenaline on the acquisition and maintenance of ethanol preference in a taste conditioning paradigm. *Psychopharmacology, 90*(3), 336-340.

Hamberg, J. M., & Spear, N. E. (1978). Alleviation of forgetting of discrimination learning. *Learning and Motivation, 9,* 466-476.

Hartshorn, K., Rovee-Collier, C., Gerhardstein, P., Bhatt, R. S., Wondoloski, T. L., Klein, P., Gilch, J., Wurtzel, N., & Campos-de-Carvalho, M. (1998). The ontogeny of long-term memory over the first year-and-a-half of life. *Developmental Psychobiology, 32*, 69-89.

Hill, D. J., Hogg, J., Petrik, J., Arany, E., & Han, V. K. (1999). Cellular distribution and ontogeny of insulin-like growth factors (IGFs) and IGF binding protein messenger RNAs and peptides in developing rat pancreas. *Journal of Endocrinology, 160,* 305-317.

Hill, W. L., Borovsky, D., & Rovee-Collier, C. (1988). Continuities in infant memory development. *Developmental Psychobiology, 21,* 43-62.

Howe, M. L., & Courage, M. L. (1993). On resolving the enigma of infantile amnesia. *Psychological Bulletin, 113*(2), 305-326.

Introini-Collison, I. B., & McGaugh, J. L. (1991). Interaction of hormones and neurotransmitter systems in the modulation of memory storage. In R. C. A. Frederickson, J. L. McGaugh, & D. L. Felten (Eds.). *Peripheral signaling of the brain: Role in neural-immune interactions and learning and memory* (pp. 275-301). Ashland, OH: Hogrefe & Huber Publishers.

Izquierdo, I., Barcik, N. R., & Brioni, J. D. (1989). Pretest β-endorphin and epinephrine, but not oxotremorine, reverse retrograde interference of a conditioned emotional response in mice. *Pharmacology, Biochemistry, and Behavior, 33*(3), 545-548.

Izquierdo, I., & Pereira, M. E. (1989). Post-training memory facilitation blocks extinction but not retroactive interference. *Behavioral & Neural Biology, 51*(1), 108-113.

Kirby, R. H. (1963). Acquisition, extinction, and retention of an avoidance response in rats as a function of age. *Journal of Comparative and Physiological Psychology, 56,* 158-162.

Koob, G. F., Lebrun, C., Bluthe, R. M., Dantzer, R., Dorsa, D. M., & Le Moal, M. (1991). Vasopressin and learning: Peripheral and central mechanisms. In R. C. A. Frederickson, J. L. McGaugh, & D. L. Felten (Eds.), *Peripheral signaling and the brain: Role in neural-immune interactions and learning and memory* (pp. 351-363). Lewiston, NY: Hogrefe & Huber.

Levine, S. (1994). The ontogeny of the hypothalamic-pituitary-adrenal axis. The influence of maternal factors. *Annals of the New York Academy of Science, 746,* 275-293.

Liang, K. C., McGaugh, J. L., & Yao, H. Y. (1990). Involvement of amygdala pathways in the influence of post-training intra-amygdala norepinephrine and peripheral epinephrine on memory storage. *Brain Research, 508*(2), 225-233.

Lu, R. B., Lebenthal, E., & Lee, P. C. (1987). Developmental changes of glucocorticoid receptors in the rat pancreas. *Journal of Steroid Biochemistry, 26,* 213-218.

McGaugh, J. L. (1983). Hormonal influences on memory. *Annual Review of Psychology, 34,* 297-323.

Mcgaugh, J. L., & Roozendaal, B. (2002). Role of adrenal stress hormones in forming lasting memories in the brain. *Current Opinion in Neurobiology, 12*(2), 205-210.

Miyashita, T., & Williams, C. L. (2004). Peripheral arousal-related hormones modulate norepinephrine release in the hippocampus via influences on brainstem nuclei. *Behavioural Brain Research, 153,* 87-95.

Morley, J. E. & Flood, J. F. (1991). Gut peptides as modulators of memory. In R. C. A. Frederickson, J. L. McGaugh, & D. L. Felten (Eds.), *Peripheral signaling of the brain: Role in neural-immune interactions and learning and memory* (pp. 379-387). Lewiston, NY: Hogrefe & Huber.

Nordby, T., Torras-Garcia, M., Portell-Cortes, I., & Costa-Miserachs, D. (2006). Posttraining epinephrine treatment reduces the need for extensive training. *Physiology & Behavior, 89*, 718-723.

Pillemer, D. B., & White, S. H. (1989). Childhood events recalled by children and adults. In H. W. Reese (Ed.), *Advances in child development and behavior*, Vol. 21 (pp. 297-340). Orlando, FL: Academic Press.

Richardson, R., Wang, P., & Campbell, B. A. (1993). Reactivation of nonassociative memory. *Developmental Psychobiology, 26,* 1-23.

Rovee-Collier, C. K., & Hayne, H. (1987). Reactivation of infant memory: Implications for cognitive development. In H. W. Reese (Ed.), *Advances in child development and behavior* (Vol. 20, pp. 185-238). San Diego, CA: Academic Press.

Rovee-Collier, C. K., Sullivan, M. W., Enright, M., Lucas, D., & Fagan, J. W. (1980). Reactivation of infant memory. *Science, 208,* 1159-1161.

Schapiro, S., Geller, E., & Eiduson, S. (1962). Neonatal adrenal cortical response to stress and vasopressin. *Proceedings of Social, Experimental, and Biological Medicine, 109,* 937-941.

Schlessinger, A. R., Cowan, W. M., & gottlieb, D. I. (1975). An autoradiographic study of the time of origin and the pattern of granule cell migration in the dentate gyrus of the rat. *Journal of Comparative Neurology, 159,* 149-176.

Schmidt, M., Enthoven, L., van der Mark, M., Levine, S., de Kloet, E. R., & Oitzl, M. S. (2003). The postnatal development of the hypothalamic-pituitary-adrenal axis in the mouse. *International Journal of Developmental Neuroscience, 21,* 125-132.

Sheingold, K., & Tenney, Y. (1982). Memory for a salient childhood event. In U. Neisser (Ed.), *Memory observed: Remembering in natural contexts*. San Francisco, CA: Freeman.

Silvers, J. M., Harrod, S. B., Ferris, M. J., Mactutus, C. F., & Booze, R. M. (2006). Automation of the novel object recognition task [Abstract]. *Society for Neuroscience, 751.6.*

Spear, N. E., & Parsons, P. J. (1976). Analysis of a reactivation treatment: Ontogenetic determinants of alleviated forgetting. In D. L. Medin, W. A. Roberts, & R. T. Davis (Eds.), *Processes of animal memory* (pp. 135-165). Hillsdale, NJ: Lawrence Erlbaum.

Spear, N. E., & Riccio, D. C. (1994). *Memory, phenomena, and principles*. Boston, MA: Allyn and Bacon.

Spear, N. E., & Rudy, J. W. (1991). Test of ontogeny of learning and memory: Issues, methods, and results. In H. N. Shair, G. A. Barr, & M. A. Hofer (Eds.), *Developmental psychobiology: New methods and changing concepts.* New York, NY: Oxford University Press.

Steckler, T., Drinkenburg, W. H., Sahgal, A., & Aggleton, J. P. (1998). Recognition memory in rats – I. Concepts and classification. *Progress in Neurobiology, 54*(3), 289-311.

Steptoe, A. (1987). The assessment of sympathetic nervous function in human stress research. *Journal of Psychosomatic Research, 31*(2), 141-152.

Sternberg, D. B., Isaacs, K. R., Gold, P. E., & McGaugh, J. L. (1985). Epinephrine facilitation of appetitive learning: Attenuation with adrenergic receptor antagonists. *Behvioral & Neural Biology, 44*(3), 447-453.

Usher, J. A., & Neisser, U. (1993). Childhood amnesia and the beginnings of memory for four early life events. *Journal of Experimental Psychology: General, 122,* 155-165.

Vannucci, S. J. (1994). Developmental expression of GLUT1 and GLUT3 glucose transporters in rat brain. *Journal of Neurochemistry, 62,* 240-246.

Vannucci, S. J., Clark, R. R., Koehler-Stec, E., Li, K., Smith, C. B., Davies, P., Maher, F., & Simpson, I. A. (1998). Glucose transporter expression in brain: Relationship to cerebral glucose utilization. *Developmental Neuroscience, 20,* 369-379.

Vannucci, S. J., Seaman, L. B., Brucklacher, R. M., & Vannucci, R. C. (1994). Glucose transport in developing rat brain glucose transporter proteins, rate constants, and cerebral glucose utilization. *Molecular and Cellular Biochemistry, 140,* 177-184.

Vannucci, S. J., & Simpson, I. A. (2003). Developmental switch in brain nutrient transporter expression in the rat. *American Journal of Physiology, 48,* E1127-E1134.

Vannucci, S. J., Willing, L. B., & Vannucci, R. C. (1993). Developmental expression of glucose transporters, GLUT1 and GLUT3, in postnatal rat brain. *Advances in Experimental and Medical Biology, 331,* 3-7.

Vazquez, D. M. (1998). Stress and the developing limbic-hypothalamic-pituitary-adrenal axis. *Psychoneuroendocrinology, 23*(7), 663-700.

Williams, C. L., & McGaugh, J. L. (1993). Reversible lesions of the nucleus of the solitary tract attenuate the memory-modulating effects of posttraining epinephrine. *Behavioral Neuroscience, 107*(6), 955-962.

Williams, C. L., Men, D., & Clayton, E. C. (2000). The effects of noradrenergic activation of the nucleus tractus solitarius on memory and in potentiating norepinephrine release in the amygdala. *Behavioral Neuroscience, 114*(6), 1131-1144.

Williams, C. L., Men, D., Clayton, E. C., & Gold, P. E. (1998). Norepinephrine release in the amygdala after systemic injection of epinephrine or escapable footshock: Contribution of the nucleus of the solitary tract. *Behavioral Neuroscience, 112*(6), 1414-1422.

Reviewed by Matthew Anderson, Ph.D., Saint Joseph's University

In: Research Progress on Epinephrine
Editors: A. G. Lawson and R. I. Gorman, pp. 43-58
ISBN: 978-1-60456-443-3

Chapter II

Epinephrine Overview in the Heart

Mitsuhiro Isaka
Pediatric Cardiac Surgery, Arkansas Children's Hospital,
800 Marshall Street, Slot677, Little Rock, AR 72202, USA

Abstract

Cardiac diseases are frequent causes of morbidity and mortality all over the world which signify a major priority field in medical research. However, a significant improvement has been made during last decades in diagnosis and therapy of cardiac diseases, which invites the need for better understanding of their pathophysiological basis. Many neurohormoral changes occur as a consequence of the hemodynamic alternations in cardiac diseases, of which increased sympathetic nervous modulation is likely to be detrimental to cardiac diseases. Epinephrine (Epi) has the sophisticated cross-talk with some physiological substances, the critical involvement in the cardiac regulation in both health and diseases, and the adapted effect to stress. Although about ninety percent of major origins for Epi are from adrenal medulla, much less is known about extra-adrenal tissues. The origin of such extra-adrenal epinephrine stores has been explained by neuronal uptake, neuronal synthesis, synthesis by extra-adrenal chromaffin cells and neuroendocrine cells. Phenylethanolamine N-methyltransferase (PNMT), an enzyme involved in Epi synthesis, is widely distributed not only in adrenal gland but also in other organs. In heart, the PNMT is localized not mainly in intrinsic cardiac adrenergic system, but might also be in cardiomyocytes, suggesting the presence of Epi system in heart. Hence the development of knowledge for Epi in heart would extend further our knowledge in understanding cardiac diseases.

Introduction

Epinephrine (Epi), often referred to as adrenaline, was found as an important physiological substance in human body [12]. The research focused on various roles and production of Epi, has been developing after this amazing investigation.

Cardiac diseases are one of the most important diseases all over the world, which is still hot research field. However, a significant improvement has been made during last decades in cardiac diseases, which need further understanding of their pathophysiological basis. Many cardiac diseases activate the sympathetic nervous, might be likely to be detrimental to cardiac diseases. Norepinephrine (NE) is the main catecholamine released from sympathetic nerve terminals, however, Epi also has the sophisticated cross-talk with some physiological substances, the critical involvement in the cardiac regulation in both health and diseases, and the adapted effect to stress. In general, Epi has a positive chronotropic, dromotropic, inotropic, and lusotropic effects, however, Epi still has various interesting roles. Hence the development of knowledge for Epi in heart would extend further our knowledge in understanding cardiac diseases.

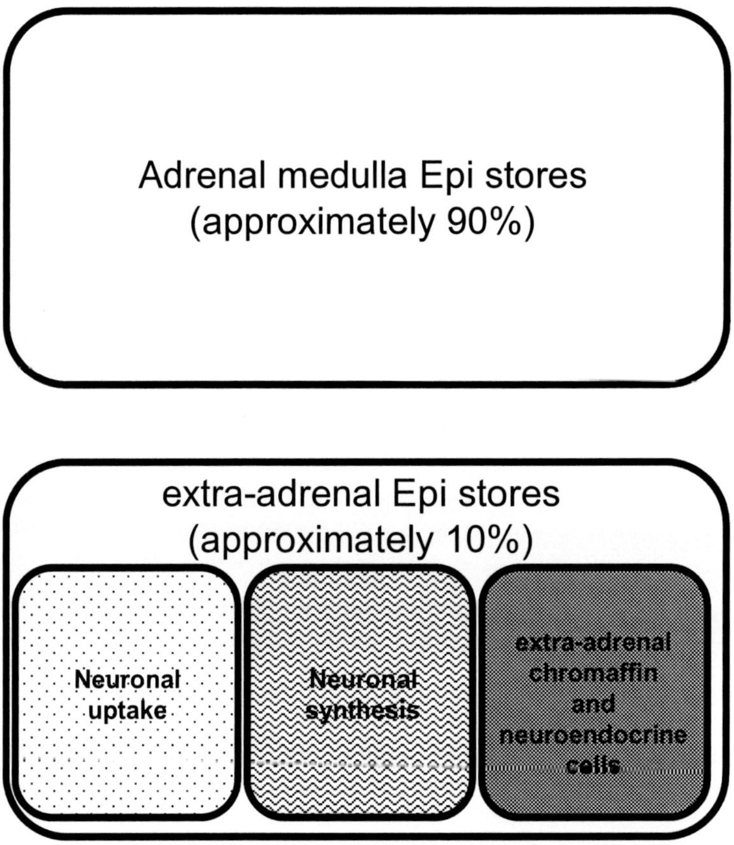

Figure 1. Epi Stores.

Epinephrine Synthesis in the Heart

Many investigators recognized major origins for Epi are adrenal medulla in human body [5, 32, 110], because approximately ninety percent of major origins for Epi are from adrenal medulla [22]. Interestingly, Epi is present in human plasma and urine after bilateral adrenalectomy [92, 111], suggesting the extra-adrenal Epi release. To address this concern, many investigators researched about the Epi origin of extra-adrenal medulla. The origin of such extra adrenal Epi stores is more controversial, however, has variously been explained by neuronal uptake of circulating Epi, neuronal epinephrine synthesis, synthesis by extra-adrenal chromaffin cells and neuroendocrine cells [64, 84, 99] (Figure 1).

Phenylethanolamine N-methyltransferase (PNMT) and nonspecific N-methyltransferase (NMT), enzymes involved in Epi synthesis, are widely distributed in human tissues, including adrenal medulla [2] and heart [2, 104]. Atria contain mainly PNMT, whereas ventricles contain both PNMT and NMT in rat heart [23]. In heart, the PNMT is localized not mainly in intrinsic cardiac adrenergic system, but might also be in cardiomyocytes, suggesting the presence of Epi system in heart. Recent data showed PNMT might be localized mainly in intrinsic cardiac adrenergic cells (ICA) or in extra-neuronal cells [42, 51], and the synthesis of Epi might be influenced by glucocorticoid and thyroid hormones [54, 56].

Epinephrine Release from the Heart

NE is main cathecolamine released from cardiac sympathetic nerve terminals, however, there are some documents about the Epi release from heart. During electrical stimulation of cardiac sympathetic nerves, Epi concentration in the coronary sinus could be increased, suggesting endogenous tissue epinephrine can act as a contrasmitter of sympathetic nerves [72]. In porcine heart, Epi release from cardiac sympathetic neurons, but they do not provide evidence that Epi augments cardiac sympathoneural NE release under basal conditions or during sympathetic activation [61]. Also, human heart could release Epi in vivo [25, 26, 27].

Tissue Epi, originated from the adrenal medulla, is released locally along with NE, mediating physiological and pathophysiological autoregulatory feedback mechanisms for further release of Epi [35, 75, 76]. In addition, the release of Epi could be modulated with various presynaptic receptors [35, 71]. Neuronal Epi release of the degree found would be sufficient to facilitate NE release, augmenting sympathetically-mediated cardiovascular responses [25, 26]. However, the cross-talk mechanism of Epi release remains unclear.

Epinephrine in Cardiovascular Regulation

The role of Epi in normal cardiovascular function remains unclear. In humans, resting plasma Epi levels are usually <80 pg/mL, apparently below the threshold at which they influence heart rate (HR) and blood pressure (BP) [11]. The abolition of Epi release by adrenal medullectomy has no detectable effect in resting humans [41], but the cardiovascular effects of adrenal medullectomy are controversial in various animal models [37, 39, 7, 63, 85].

On the other hand, the release of Epi from the adrenal medulla is among the first responses to many stressors, including dynamic exercise [3, 83, 103]. As a major stress hormone, this blood-borne Epi is involved in regulating cardiovascular function during exercise. However, because of the simultaneous release of other hormones and neurotransmitters, especially NE from sympathetic nerves, it remains unclear whether Epi plays a primary role in the cardiovascular response to exercise or even if its role is stimulatory or inhibitory in nature, despite many exercise studies in medullectomized and/or denervated animals [1, 15, 37].

In the Epi-deficient mouse model (PNMT knocked out: KO), suggesting that Epi is required for normal blood pressure and cardiac filling responses to stress but is not required for tachycardia during stress or normal cardiovascular function at rest [6]. Central adrenergic neurons generally are thought to decrease sympathetic outflow by releasing Epi on preganglionic sympathetic neurons. However, the loss of Epi in PNMT KO mice did not significantly change sympathetic activity, suggesting that central Epi does not have critical role in maintaining overall sympathetic tone and cardiovascular function at rest.

On the other hand, Epi is also well known to regulate vascular tone by stimulating the peripheral beta2-adrenergic receptors, resulting in the decrease of BP [38, 62]. Interestingly, physiological concentrations of plasma Epi decrease vascular resistance in humans [30]. In addition to circulating Epi, Epi also is synthesized in endothelial cells of blood vessels [97]. Thus, Epi may regulate vascular tone and BP locally. Vasodilation by Epi and metabolic byproducts are both thought to play a role in limiting the BP increase during exercise [9, 94]. Beta2-adrenergic receptor KO mice also have a normal basal resting BP and become hypertensive during exercise [10]. Taken together, these observations suggest that Epi-induced vasodilation is required to prevent BP overshoot during exercise but plays only a minimal role in maintaining BP at rest.

In addition to the beta2-adrenergic receptor, Epi has a potent effects via cardiac alpha and beta1 receptors, and also potent effects to constrict veins in vivo, mobilizing blood from the venous compartment and augmenting central venous pressure by decreasing venous compliance [20, 86, 95, 107, 115]. Also intravenous infusion of Epi increases HR and CO in humans [28, 30]. In addition, Epi synthesis in the heart has been associated with the development of pacemaking and cardiac conduction in recent studies [18, 19]. However, total loss of Epi in PNMT KO mice had little influence on resting cardiac function, including HR, EF, and Co in rest

In summary, Epi deficiency has no impact on basal cardiovascular functions such as HR, BP, EF, and CO. However, the exaggerated BP response to exercise and reduced cardiac filling with restraint found in our PNMT KO mice indicate that Epi is required for maintaining normal cardiovascular function during stress. The adrenal Epi response to various stressors is reduced with aging [90], and the salutary effects of Epi on cardiovascular adaptation to acute stress, as revealed here, might partly explain decreased cardiovascular homeostasis with stress in advancing age [65]. The PNMT KO mouse will allow more thorough studies involving different types of stressors (such as induced heart failure) and longitudinal studies (eg, chronic stress) to further clarify the role of Epi in cardiovascular adaptation to stress.

Epinephrine in Heart Failure

Heart failure is a major medical problem, and activates a number of neurohormonal processes in the pathophysiology [21, 59, 98, 101, 108, 112]. In approximately 50 years ago, Epi on myocardium was significantly increased in cases of fresh myocardial infarction, in congestive heart failure, and in renal uremia. It is believed that the hypoxiating action of excess Epi in the heart muscle constitutes an important pathogenic factor in the origin of certain forms of functional and degenerative heart disease [75, 76].

Epi may participate in the development of increased sympathetic nerve activity associated with high mortality in congestive heart failure [101]. The activation of the sympathetic nervous system in patients with heart failure, specifically the cardiac sympathetic nerves, thus, Epi may contribute to the poor prognosis associated with severe heart failure [52]. A high level of neuronal Epi release in heart failure could facilitate release of the major neurotransmitter NE [29]. Furthermore, nonadrenal tissues may contribute significantly to the whole body Epi release rate in heart failure and that this may arise from a site other than sympathetic neurons in heart failure [51, 52].

Another study, cardiorenal Epi release was found in patients with congestive heart failure and renal Epi release in hypertensive patients. Furthermore, Epi is removed by neuronal uptake in both the heart and kidney, and cardiac Epi spillover increases during exercise [48]. However, the role of released Epi from extra-adrenal origins in heart failure, is still not totally understood.

Epinephrine in Cardiomyopathies

Cardiomyopathes, like a hypertrophied, dilated or restrictive, are common causes for heart failure, especially the patients with dilated cardiomyopathy (DCM) needs heart transplantation.

Neurohormonal substances, such as such as Epi, NE, human atrial natriuretic peptide (hANP), could be activated in cardiomyopathies [36, 68]. In experimental and clinical studies, there are a lot of evidences that myocardial and plasms levels of Epi and NE could be elevated in DCM and hypertrophic cardiomyopathy (HCM) [49, 50, 91, 113]. However, the pathophysiological role of myocardial EPi in cardiomyopathies is still not completely understood.

Epinephrine in Myocardial Infarction

Many clinical studies showed cathecolamines have the important role in myocardial infarction (MI). Thus, sympathetic nervous system and myocardial ischemia are related bidirectionally. Activation of the sympathoadrenal system expressed as increased levels of circulating catecholamines, Epi and NE may accelerate the development of ischemic heart disease (IHD), on the other, acute myocardial infarction (AMI) may lead to activation of the sympathoadrenal system [4, 79, 96]. Increased levels of circulating catecholamines could occur in overall stage of AMI [36, 80, 81]. In addition, high amounts of NE are released from the sympathetic nerve terminals of the heart [80, 81] and massive accumulation of NE occurs in the extracellular space of the ischemic area [89]. The release is determined by local energy exhaustion and occurs in overall with the development of membrane defects within the ischemic are in which the sympathetic neurons progressively deplete from NE [82, 87].

There is one interested report about Epi in MI experimental animal model. Four weeks after MI (conronary artery ligation rat model), plasma and ventriclar (left and right) Epi, unlike NE, were markedly increased. Whereas plasma cathcholamine (Epi and NE) levels were increased 8 weeks after MI, NE concentration in the left ventricle was unchanged but Epi concentration was increased. However, the right ventricle showed an increased level of both NE and Epi 8 weeks after MI. Thus, differential changes in the status of sympathetic nerves in the left and right ventricles might be present; sympathetic activity is increased only in the left ventricle, whereas the right ventricle may play an adaptive role by increasing cathecholamine stores during the development of heart failure [31]. Taken together, Epi likely seems to have the association with time-dependent and/or region-dependent roles in MI.

Epinephrine in Myocardial Ishemia-Reperfusion

Cathecolamines are elevated by ischemia, and induces post ischemic myocardiac injury. Protracted myocardial ischemia induces much greater release of NE from cardiac sympathetic nerve terminals, than normal conditions. In this case, excessive NE release is carrier-mediated release rather than exocytosis, which could be modulated by various physiological substances, like endothlin, bradykinin, or histamine [40, 45, 46, 88].

Interestingly, there are few reports Epi under cardiac ischemia and reperfusion. Prolonged myocardial ischemia is associated with a progressive increase of Epi concentrations in the myocardial interstitial fluid [60]. PNMT, the enzyme that synthesizes Epi from NE in the adrenal gland, is present in extra-adrenal tissues including heart. Also, ischemia evokes an excessive NE accumulation in the myocardial interstitial spaces. Therefore, cardiac PNMT activity with high NE levels may contribute to cardiac epinephrine synthesis and release evoked by ischemia.

To address this question, Kuroko Y et al recently demonstrated elevated NE levels in the myocardial interstitial space [58]. The research on the relationship between catecholamine and cardiac ischemia, has been focused on NE until now. However, cardiac ischemia can induce NE release, and also Epi release from heart, in other words, local Epi in heart might have associated with cardiac ischemia, leading to cardiac dysfunctions.

Epinephrine in Development of Heart

Although it is well known the cardiovascular regulations of Epi, Epi is also preserved throughout vertebrate evolution, thus, it has been recognized the role of Epi might be important in the development of heart for several years.

Recent evidence suggests that the mammalian heart may be a source of catecholamines at early developmental stages, PNMT and other enzymes of catecholamine systhesis in fetal heart may produce low levels of Epi prior to formation of the fetal adrenal medulla because [42]. Thus, Epi synthesis has been detected in the embryonic heart before either sympathetic innervation of the heart or production of Epi in adrenal chromaffin cells [17-19, 42]. In rats, for example, the Epi biosynthetic enzyme PNMT is expressed in the heart as early as embryonic day 9.5 (E9.5), whereas the earliest appearance of this enzyme in the adrenal gland does not occur until E15.5 to E16.5 [17, 102]. Similarly, sympathetic nerves do not appear in the developing rat heart until R16 to E17 [93]. Parasympathetic innovation of the heart occurs much earlier than sympathetic innervatin but does not begin to appear until E12 in the rat. Studies with chic and human embryos have likewise demonstrated the expression of catecholamine biosynthetic enzymes in the heart before sympathetic inneravation [42-44]. Thus, the embryonic heart seems to have the capability of producing catecholamines at stages of development that precede production of catecholamines in the adrenal gland and cardiac sympathetic nerves.

Although chromaffin-like and small intensely fluorescent catecholaminergic cells have been found in and around adult hearts from many species, [13, 14, 24, 47, 69], typically in association with cardiac nerves, few studies have examined catecholamine production in the prenatal heart. These developments are via intrinsic cardiac adrenegic cells [19].

Cardiac PNMT develops early in the fetal heart and is found in relatively high levels in the adult left atrium. Intrinsic cardiac adrenergic cells are distributed throughut the adult myocardium and contain all the enzymes necessary for Epi synthesis, affected by glucocorticoid [55]. Although PNMT gene promoter region contains a glucocorticoid response region, the initial development of brain and cardiac fetal PNMT is glucocorticoid independent [116].

Epinephrine in Heart Transplantation

Heart transplantation (HTx) is a well-established treatment for patients in end stage heart failure suffered from various heart diseases. One of the primary causes of early death after HTx is cardiac graft dysfunction, suggesting that early survival is influenced by preservation and implantation injury. Recently, heart rate variability (HRV), which is characterized by a nearly fixed pattern, might be caused by the graft denervation during HTx [77]. HRV provides both independent and additional prognostic information with respect to the risk 'cardiac mortality or deterioration of congestive heart failure [57].

As a consequence of the denervation, heart function and activity depend predominantly on hemodynamic loading conditions (preload and afterload) and circulating catecholamines. Myocardial NE is markedly reduced after HTx because of interruption of postganglionic cardiac sympathetic nerves, thus, one of the suspected alternatives of cardiac regulation in this situation is autonomous production of Epi in the myocardium. In vivo experimental model, myocardial NE and Epi are depleted in all portions of shot-term autotransplanted canine hearts [66, 74]. In long-term autotransplanted canine hearts about 50% of control NE and Epi are found [66, 74]. Dopamine content, however, is only modestly decreased in short- and long-term autotransplanted canine hearts [16, 66]. In the transplanted human heart, myocardial catecholamines (NE, Epi and dopamine) were undetectable in short-term HTx patients, and also in long-term HTx patients. However, there were the low myocardial NE levels with significant elevated levels of Epi in some patients, suggesting that the sympathetic response probably depends on variations in plasma catecholamines or cardiac beta-receptor density [78]. However, further evidence will be needed to discuss the role of Epi in HTx.

Numerous studies of HRV documented the possibility of reinevation late after HTx, dominantly of the sympathetic part [8, 53]. Although an apparent evidence of the possibility of the graft reinervation is the sensation of anginal chest pain by some patients with graft coronary artery vasculopathy, HRV might be associated with Epi. HTx interrupts the afferent and efferent innervations of the graft, thus cardiac renervation is very important to maintain cardiac contractility heart rate and so on. To be regretting things, there are only two reports about PNMT before and after HTx [33, 34], suggesting the association with cardiac re-inervation after HTx.

Epinephrine in Arrhythmia

Epi has been a mainstay of resuscitation therapy for more than 100 years; however, its use increases myocardial oxygen consumption and the drug has arrhythmogenic effects. Epi in physiologic concentrations shortens the effective refractory period of the atrium, atrioventricular (AV) node and ventricle, improves AV node conduction and may facilitate the induction of sustained ventricular tachycardia [67]. In addition, Epi released during ventricular tachycardia (VT) or early fibrillation (VF) appears to be instrumental in stabilizing fibrillation [73, 109].

Although there are a lot of report about Epi on arrhythmias, such as ventricular fibriliation (VF) and long QT syndrome (LQTS) [70, 100, 105], mechanism of Epi arrhythmogenic effects remain unclear. Clinical studies suggest that Epi facilitates ventricular fibrillation (VF) although mechanisms remain unclear. Epi reduced fibrillation, and also reduced the probability of spontaneous termination of VF during early stage. In addition, Epi significanthy decreased mean fibrillation cycle length and mean action potential duration. These suggest that Epi increases the probability of VF induction and decreases the probability of spontaneous defibrillation [106].

The mechanisms that may lead to cardiac arrhythmias, have been studies in atrial and ventricular tissues from human hearts. For instance, in human atrial fibers, diastolic depolarization (DD), which modifies the recovery of premature action potentials, was consistently present, but did not induce spontaneous discharge. Human ventricular fibers did not exhibit DD and were more resistant to calcium ion overload [114]. Thus, in atrial tissues the presence of DD may not induce automatic arrhymias, but it may influence conduction and re-entry rhythms. Interestingly, subsequent administration of Epi provoked both bradycardia-dependent early afterdepolarizations (EADs) and tachycardia-dependent delayed afterdepolarization (DADs). In clofilium-treated purkinje fibers, with predominantly EADs observed in d, l-sotanol-treated purkinje fibers, it seems like the facilitation of Epi-induced EADs and DADs by class III antiarrhythmic drugs [70]. Also, Epi enhanced DD, could induce delayed after depolarizations (DADs) and trigger repetitive activity [114].

Summary

Epi has various important effects in heart, thus a local Epi system in heart has very important and/or unique roles in cardiovascular regulations and pathophysiology. Although Epi is one of the most well-known neurohormonal substances, the effect and mechanism of Epi remain unclear. In addition, further studies will be needed, for developing the knowledge and understanding the role of Epi,

References

[1] Ashkar E, & Hamilton WF. (1963) Cardiovascular response to graded exercise in the sympathectomized-vagotomized dog. *Am J Physiol.* 1963 204: 291-296.

[2] Axelrod J. (1962) Purification and properties of phenylethanolamine-N-methyl transferase. *J Biol Chem*. 237: 1657-1660.

[3] Axelrod J, & Reisine TD. (1984) Stress hormones: their interaction and regulation. *Science*. 224: 452-459.

[4] Bacaner M, Brietenbucher J, & LaBree J. (2004) Prevention of ventricular fibrillation, acute myocardial infarction (myocardial necrosis), heart failure, and mortality by bretylium: is ischemic heart disease primarily adrenergic cardiovascular disease? *Am J Ther*. 11: 366-411.

[5] Badder EM, Santen R, Samojlik E, & Harrison TS. (1980) Adrenal medullary epinephrine secretion: effects of cortisol alone and combined with aminoglutethimide. *J Lab Clin Med*. 96: 815-821.

[6] Bao X, Lu CM, Liu F, Gu Y, Dalton ND, Zhu BQ, Foster E, Chen J, Karliner JS, Ross J Jr, Simpson PC, & Ziegler MG. (2007) Epinephrine is required for normal cardiovascular responses to stress in the phenylethanolamine N-methyltransferase knockout mouse. *Circulation*. 116: 1024-1031.

[7] Bao G, Metreveli N, Li R, Taylor A, & Fletcher EC. (1997) Blood pressure response to chronic episodic hypoxia: role of the sympathetic nervous system. *J Appl Physiol.* 83: 95-101.

[8] Bengel FM, Ueberfuhr P, Hesse T, Schiepel N, Ziegler SI, Scholz S, Nekolla SG, Reichart B, & Schwaiger M. (2002) Clinical determinations of ventricular sympathetic reinervation after orthotopic heart transplantation. *Circulation.* 106: 831-835.

[9] Celander O. (1954) The range of control exercised by the sympathico-adrenal system; a quantitative study on blood vessels and other smooth muscle effectors in the cat. *Acta Physiol Scand.* 32 (suppl): 1-132.

[10] Chruscinski AJ, Rohrer DK, Schauble E, Desai KH, Bernstein D, & Kobilka BK. (1999) Targeted distruption of the beta2 adrenergic receptor gene. *J Biol Chem.* 274: 16694-16700.

[11] Clutter WE, Bier DM, Shah SD, & Cryer PE. (1980) Epinephrine plasma metabolic clearance rates and physiologic thresholds for metabolic and hemodynamic actions in man. *J Clin Invest.* 66: 94-101.

[12] Cori CF. (1929) The rate of absorption of epinephrine from the subcutaneous tissue. *Science.* 70: 355-356.

[13] Cottle MK. (1984) Distribution of catecholamine-containing cells in the atrial region in rats and ground squirrels. *Histochem J.* 16: 1137-1146.

[14] Dail WGJ, & Palmer GC. (1973) Localization and correlation of catecholamine containing cells with adenyl cyclase and phosphodiesterase activities in the human fetal heart. *Anat Rec.* 177: 265-287.

[15] Donald DE, & Shepherd JT. (1963) Response to exercise in dogs with cardiac denervation. *Am J Physiol.* 205: 393-400.

[16] Drake AJ, & Stanford C. (1982) Effect of cardiac denervation on catecholamine levels in dog heart. *J Physiol.* 324: 14P.

[17] Ebert SN, Baden JM, Mathers LH, Siddall BJ, & Wong DL.(1996) Expression of phenylethanolamine n-methyltransferase in the embryonic rat heart. *J Mol Cell Cardiol.*28: 1653-1658.

[18] Ebert SN, Rong Q, Boe S, Thompson RP, Grinberg A, & Pfeifer K.(2004) argeted insertion of the Cre-recombinase gene at the phenylethanolamine n-methyltransferase locus: a new model for studying the developmental distribution of adrenergic cells. *Dev Dyn.* 231: 849-858.

[19] Ebert SN, & Thompson RP. (2001) Embryonic epinephrine synthesis in the rat heart before innervation: association with pacemaking and conduction tissue development. *Circ Res.* 88: 117-124.

[20] Eckstein JW, & Hamilton WK. (1957) The pressure-volume responses of human forearm veins during epinephrine and norepinephrine infusions. *J Clin Invest.* 36: 1663-1671.

[21] Edvinsson L, Ekman R, Hedner P, & Valdemarsson S. (1990) Congestive heart failure: involvement of perivascular peptides reflecting activity in sympathetic, parasympathetic and afferent fibers. *Eur J Clin Invest.* 20: 85-89.

[22] Eisenhofer G, Rundquist B, Aneman A, Friberg P, Dakak N, Kopin IJ, Jacobs MC, & Lenders JW. (1995) Regional release and removal of catecholamines and extraneuronal metabolism to metanephrines. *J Clin Endocrinol Metab*. 80: 3009-3017.

[23] Elayan H, Kennedy BP, & Ziegler MG. (1990) Cardiac atria and ventricles contain different inducible adrenaline synthesizing enzymes. *Cardiovasc Res*. 24: 53-56.

[24] Ellison JP, & Hibbs RG. (1974) Catecholamine-containing cells of the guinea pig heart: an ultrastructual study. *J Mol Cell Cardiol*. 6: 17-26.

[25] Esler M, Eisenhofer G, Chin J, Jennings G, Meredith I, Cox H, Lambert G, Thompson J, & Dart A. (1991) Is adrenaline released by sympathetic nerves in man? *Clin Auton Res*. 1: 103-108.

[26] Esler M, Eisenhofer G, Dart A, Chin J, Cox H, Lambert G, & Jennings G. (1991) Adrenaline release by the human heart. *Clin Exp Pharmacol Physiol*. 18:67-70.

[27] Esler M, Kaye D, Thompson J, Jennings G, Cox H, Turner A, Lambert G, & Seals D. (1995) Effects of aging on epinephrine secretion and regional release of epinephrine from the human heart. *J Clin Endocrinol Metab*. 80: 435-442.

[28] Fellows IW, Bennett T, & MacDonald IA. (1985) The effect of adrenaline upon cardiovascular and metabolic functions in man. *Clin Sci*. 69: 215-222.

[29] Floras JS. (1992) Epinephrine and the genesis of hypertension. *Hypertension Dallas*. 19: 1-18.

[30] Freyschuss U, Hjemdahl P, Juhlin-Dannfelt A, & Linde B. (1986) cardiovascular and metabolic responses to low dose adrenaline infusion: an invasive study in humans. *Clin Sci (Lond)*. 70: 199-206.

[31] Ganguly PK, Dhalla KS, Shao Q, Beamish RE, & Dhalla NS. (1997) Differential changes in sympathetic activity in left and right ventricules in congestive heart failure after myocardial infarction. *Am Heart J*. 133: 340-345.

[32] Goldenberg M, Faber M, Alston EJ, & Chargaff EC. (1949) Evidence for the occurrence of norepinephrine in the adrenal medulla. *Science*. 109: 534-535.

[33] Goncalvesova E, Krizanova O, Micutkova L, Mravec B, Ksinantova L, Fabian J, & Kvernansky R. (2005) Phenylethanolamine N-methyltransferase gene expression in transplanted human heart. *Transplant Proceed*. 37: 1340-1342.

[34] Goncalvesova E, Micutkova L, Mravec B, Ksinantova L, Krizanova O, Fabian J, & Kvetnansky R. (2004) Changes in gene expression of phenylethanolamine N-methyltransferase in the transplanted human heart. *Ann N.Y. Acad. Sci*. 1018: 430-436.

[35] Goshima Y, Kubo T, & Misu Y. (1985) Autoregulation of endogenous epinephrine release via presynaptic adrenoceptors in the rat hypothalamic slice. *J Pharmacol and Exper Therapeu*. 235: 248-253.

[36] Hara H, Ogihara T, Nakamaru M, Rakugi H, & Tateyama H. (1988) Changes in the levels of plasma atrial natriuretic peptide, hemodynamic measurements, and the levels of vasoactive hormones during the clinical course of congestive heart failure. *Clin Cardiol*. 11: 743-747.

[37] Harakal C, Reidenberg MM, Sevy RW, & Ohler EA. (1966) Hemodynamic effects of adrenal medullectomy in the dog. *Am J Physiol*. 210: 5-6.

[38] Hardman JG, Limbird LE, & Gilman AG. (2001) *Goodman and Gilman's The Pharmacological Basis of Therapeutics.* 10th ed. New York: McGraw-Hill Co. Inc: 210-211.

[39] Hasbak P, Peterson JS, Shalmi M, Lam HR, Christensen NJ, & Christensen S. (1995) Role of the adrenal medulla in control of blood pressure and renal function during furosemide-induced volume depletion. *J Hypertens*. 13: 235-242.

[40] Hatta E, Maruyama R, Marshall SJ, Imamura M, & Levi R. (1999) Bradykinin promotes ischemic norepinephrine release in guinea-pig and human hearts. *J Pharmacol Exerp Thearapeu*. 288: 919-927.

[41] Howlett K, Galbo H, Lorentsen J, Bergeron R, Zimmerman-Belsing T, Bulow J, Feldt-Rasmussen U, & Kjaer M. (1999) Effect of adrenaline on glucose kinetics during exercise in adrenaletomised humans. *J Physiol*. 519: 911-921.

[42] Huang MH, Friend DS, Sunday ME, Singh K, Haley K, Austen KF, Kelly RA, & Smith TW. (1996) An intrinsic adrenergic system in mammalian heart. *J Clin Invest*. 98: 1298-1303.

[43] Ignarro LJ, & Shideman FE. (1968) Appearance and concentrations of catecholamines and their biosynthesis in the embryonic and developing chick. *J Pharmacol Exp Ther*. 159: 38-48.

[44] Ignarro LJ, & Shideman FE. (1968) Norepinephrine and epinephrine in the embryo and embryonic heart of the chick: uptake and subcellular distribution. *J Pharmacol Exp Ther*. 159: 49-58.

[45] Imamura M, Lander HM, & Levi R. (1996) Activation of histamine H3-receptors inhibits carrier-mediated norepinephrine release during protracted myocardial ischemia. Comparison with adenosine A1-receptors and alpha2-adrenoceptors. *Circ Res*. 78: 475-481.

[46] Isaka M, Kudo A, Imamura M, Kawakami H, & Yasuda K. (2007) Endothelin receptors, localized in sympathetic nerve terminals of the heart, modulate norepinephrine release and reperfusion arrhythmias. *Basic Res Cardiol*. 2007 102: 154-162.

[47] Jacobowitz D. (1967) Histochemical studies of the relationship of chromaffin cells and adrenergic nerve fibers to the cardiac ganglia of several species. *J Pharmacol Exp Ther*. 158: 227-240.

[48] Johansson M, Rundqvist B, Eisenhofer G, & Friberg P. (1997) Cardiorenal epinephrine kinetics: evidence for neuronal release in the human heart. *Am J Physiol*. 273: H2178-H2185.

[49] Kanemoto N, Imaoka C, hiramatsu K, & Goto Y. (1988) A case of normotensive pheochromocytoma masquerading as a dilated cardiomyopathy. *Jpn Circ J*. 50: 1128-1132.

[50] Kawai C, Yui Y, Hoshino T, Sasayama S, & Matsumori A. (1983) Myocardial catecholamines in hypertrophic and dilated (congestive) cardiomyopathy: a biopsy study. *J Am Coll Cardiol*. 2: 834-840.

[51] Kaye DM, Lefkovits J, Cox H, Lambert G, Jennings G, Turner A, & Ester MD. (1995) Regional epinephrine kinetics in human heart failure: evidence for extra-adrenal, nonneural release. *Am J Physiol*. 269: H182-188.

[52] Kaye DM, Lefkovits J, Jennings GL, Bergin P, Broughton A, & Esler MD. (1995) Adverse consequences of high sympathetic nervous activity in the failing human heart. *J Am Coll Cardiol*. 26: 1257-1263.

[53] Keeley EC, Toth ZK, & Goldberg AD. (2000) Long-term assessment of heart rate variability in cardiac transplant recipients. *J Heart Lung transplant*. 19: 310-312.

[54] Kennedy B, Bigby TD, & Ziegler MG. (1995) Nonadrenal epinephrine-forming enzymes in humans. Characteristics, distribution, regulation, and relationship to epinephrine levels. *J Clin Invest*. 95: 2896-2902.

[55] Kennedy B, Elayan H, & Ziegler MG. (1993) Glucocorticoid hypertension and nonadrenal phenylethanolamine N-methyltransferase. *Hypertension*. 21: 415-419.

[56] Kennedy B, & Ziegler MG. (1991) Cardiac epinephrine synthesis. Regulation by a glucocorticoid. *Circulation*. 84: 891-895.

[57] Kruger C, Lahm T, Zugck C, Kell R, Schellberg D, Schweizer MW, KÜbler W, Haass M. (2002) heart rate variability enhances the prognostic value of established parameters in patients with congestive heart failure. *Z Kardiol*. 91: 1003-1012.

[58] Kuroko Y, Yamazaki T, Tokunaga N, Akiyama T, Kitagawa H, Ishino K, Sano S, & Mori H. (2007) Cardiac epinephrine synthesis and ischemia-induced myocardial epinephrine release. *Cardiovasc Res*. 2007 74: 438-444.

[59] Kurose M, Okumura K, Ogawa H, Yoshimura M, Morita E, & Yasue H. (1994) Reduced cardiac extraction of norepinephrine and epinephrine in patients with heart failure--correlation with left ventricular function. *Int J Cardiol*. 47: 21-29.

[60] Lameris TW, de Zeeuw S, Alberts G, Boomsma F, Duncker DJ, Verdouw PD, Veld AJ, & van Den Meiracker AH. (2000) Time course and mechanism of myocardial catecholamine release during transient ischemia in vivo. *Circulation*. 101: 2645-250.

[61] Lameris TW, de Zeeuw S, Duncker DJ, Tietge W, Alberts G, Boomsma F, Verdouw PD, & van den Meiracker AH. (2002) Epinephrine in the heart: uptake and release, but no facilitation of norepinephrine release. *Circulation*. 106: 860-865.

[62] Lands AM, Arnold A, McAuliff JP, Luduena FP, & Brown TG Jr. (1967) Differentiation of receptor systems activated by sympathomimetic amines. *Nature*. 214: 597-598.

[63] Lange DL, Haywood JR, & Hinojosa-Laborde C. (1998) Role of the adrenal medullae in male and female DOCA-salt hypertensive rats. *Hypertension*. 31: 403-408.

[64] Majewski H, Hedler L, & Starke K. (1982) The noradrenaline rate in the anaesthetized rabbit: facilitation by adrenaline. *Naunyn Schmiedebergs Arch Pharmacol*. 321: 20-27.

[65] Meites J. (1991) Aging studies. *Science*. 251: 855.

[66] Mohanty PK, Sowers JR, Thames MD, Beck FW, Kawaguchi A, & Lower RR. (1986) Myocardial norepinephrine, epinephrine and dopamine concentrations after cardiac autotransplantation in dogs. *J Am Coll Cardiol*. 7: 419-424.

[67] Morady F, Nelson SD, Kou WH, Pratley R, Schmaltz S, De Buitleir M, & Halter JB. (1988) Electrophysiologic effects of epinephrine in humans. *J Am Coll Cardiol*. 11: 1235-1244.

[68] Ogino K, Ogura K, Kinugawa T, Osaki S, Kato M, Furuse Y, Kinugasa Y, Tomikura Y, Igawa O, Hisatome I, & Shigemasa C. (2004) Neurohumoral profiles in patients

with hypertrophic cardiomyopathy: differences to hypertensive left ventricular hypertrophy. *Circ J.* 68: 444-450.

[69] Papka RE. (1974) A study of catecholamine-containing cells in the hearts of fetal and postnatal rabbits by fluorescence and electron microscopy. *Cell Tissue Res.* 154: 471-484.

[70] Patterson E, Scherlag BJ, Szabo B, & Lazzara R. (1997) Facilitation of epinephrine-induced afterdepolarizations by class III antiarrhythmic drugs. *J Electrocardiol.* 30: 217-224.

[71] Peronnet F, Boudreau G, Champlain JD, & Nadeau R. (1994) Effect of changes in myocardial epinephrine stores on plasma norepinephrine gradient across the dog heart. *Am J Physiol.* 266: H2404-2409.

[72] Péronnet F, Nadeau R, Boudreau G, Cardinal R, Lamontagne D, Yamaguchi N, & De Champlain J. (1988) Epinephrine release from the heart during left stellate ganglion stimulation in dogs. *Am J Physiol.* 254: R659-662.

[73] Peuhkurinen KJ, Huikuri HV, Linnaluoto M, & Takkunen JT. (1994) Changes in myocardial metabolism and transcardiac electrolytes during simulated ventricular tachycardia: effects of beta-adrenergic blockade. *Am Heart J.* 128: 96-105.

[74] Potter LT, Cooper T, Willman VL, & Wolfe DE. (1965) Synthesis, binding, release, and metabolism of norepinephrine in normal and transplanted dog hearts. *Circ Res.* 16: 468-481.

[75] Raab W, & Gigee W. (1955) Specific avidity of the heart muscle to absorb and store epinephrine and norepinephrine. *Circ Res.* 3: 553-558.

[76] Raab W, & Gigee W. (1955) Norepinephrine and epinephrine content of normal and diseased human hearts. *Circulation.* 11: 593-603.

[77] Ramaekers D, Ector H, Vanhaecke J, van Cleemput J, & van de Werf F. (1996) Heart rate variability after cardiac transplantation in humans. *Pacing Clin Electrophysiol.* 19: 2112-2119.

[78] Regitz V, Bossaller C, Strasser R, Schüler S, Hetzer R, & Fleck E. (1990) Myocardial catecholamine content after heart transplantation. *Circulation.* 82: 620-623.

[79] Remme WJ. (1998) The sympathetic nervous system and ischaemic heart disease. *Eur Heart J.* 19 (Suppl): F62-71.

[80] Remme WJ, Kruyssen DA, Look MP, Bootsma M, & de Leeuw PW. (1994) Systemic and cardiac neuroendocrine activation and severity of myocardial ischemia in humans. *J Am Coll Cardiol.* 23: 82-91.

[81] Remme WJ, de Leeuw PW, Bootsma M, Look MP, & Kruijssen DA. (1991) Systemic neurohumoral activation and vasoconstriction during pacing-induced acute myocardial ischemia in patients with stable angina pectoris. *Am J Cardiol.* 68: 181-186.

[82] Richardt G, Waas W, Kranzhöfer R, Mayer E, & Schömig A. (1987) Adenosine inhibits exocytotic release of endogenous noradrenaline in rat heart: a protective mechanism in early myocardial ischemia. *Circ Res.* 61: 117-123.

[83] Rowell LB, Brengelmann GL, & Freund PR. (1987) Unaltered norepinephrine-heart rate relationship in exercise with exogenous heat. *J Appl Physiol.* 62: 646-650.

[84] Ruggiero DA, Gatti PJ, Gillis RA, Norman WP, Anwar M, & Reis DJ. (1986) Adrenaline-synthesizing neurons in the medulla of the cat. *J Comp Neurol.* 252: 532-542.

[85] Rutter PC, Potocnik SJ, & Ludbrook J. (1987) Sympathoadrenal mechanisms in cardiovascular responses to naloxone after hemorrhage. *Am J Physiol.* 252: H40-46.

[86] Sandblom E, Axelsson M, & Farrell AP. (2006) Central venous pressure and mean circulatory filling pressure in the dogfish Squalus acanthias: adrenergic control and role of the pericardium. *Am J Physiol Regul Integr Comp Physiol.* 291: R1465-1473.

[87] Schömig A. (1988) Adrenergic mechanisms in myocardial infarction: cardiac and systemic catecholamine release. *J Cardiovasc Pharmacol.* 12 (Suppl): S1-7.

[88] Schömig A. (1990) Catecholamines in myocardial ischemia. Systemic and cardiac release. *Circulation.* 82 (Suppl): II13-22.

[89] Schömig A, Fischer S, Kurz T, Richardt G, & Schömig E. (1987) Nonexocytotic release of endogenous noradrenaline in the ischemic and anoxic rat heart: mechanism and metabolic requirements. *Circ Res.* 60: 194-205.

[90] Seals DR, & Esler MD. (2000) Human ageing and the sympathoadrenal system. *J Physiol.* 528: 407-417.

[91] Seferović PM, Maksimović R, Ostojić M, Stepanović S, Nikolić J, Vasiljević JD, Kanjuh V, Seferović D, Simeunović S, & Ristić A. (1995) Myocardial catecholamines in primary heart muscle disease: fact or fancy? *Eur Heart J.* 16 (Suppl): 124-127.

[92] Shah SD, Tse TF, Clutter WE, & Cryer PE. (1984) The human sympathochromaffin system. *Am J Physiol.* 247: E380-384.

[93] Shigenobu K, Tanaka H, & Kasuya Y. (1988) Changes in sensitivity of rat heart to norepinephrine and isoproterenol during pre- and postnatal development and its relation to sympathetic innervation. *Dev Pharmacol Ther.* 11: 226-236.

[94] Singh JP, Larson MG, Manolio TA, O'Donnell CJ, Lauer M, Evans JC, & Levy D. (1999) Blood pressure response during treadmill testing as a risk factor for new-onset hypertension. The Framingham heart study. *Circulation.* 99: 1831-1836.

[95] Skals M, Skovgaard N, Taylor EW, Leite CA, Abe AS, & Wang T. (2006) Cardiovascular changes under normoxic and hypoxic conditions in the air-breathing teleost Synbranchus marmoratus: importance of the venous system. *J Exp Biol.* 209: 4167-4173.

[96] Slavíková J, Kuncová J, & Topolcan O. (2007) Plasma catecholamines and ischemic heart disease. *Clin Cardiol.* 30: 326-330.

[97] Spatz M, Nagatsu I, Maruki C, Yoshida M, Kondo Y, & Bembry J. (1982) The presence of phenylethanolamine-N-methyltransferase in cerebral microvessel and endothelial cultures. *Brain Res.* 240: 191-194.

[98] Staroukine M, Devriendt J, Decoodt P, & Verniory A. (1984) Relationships between plasma epinephrine, norepinephrine, dopamine and angiotensin II concentrations, renin activity, hemodynamic state and prognosis in acute heart failure. *Acta Cardiol.* 39: 131-138.

[99] Sudo A. (1985) Accumulation of adrenaline in sympathetic nerve endings in various organs of the rat exposed to swimming stress. *Jpn J Pharmacol.* 38: 367-374.

[100] Sun ZH, Swan H, Viitasalo M, & Toivonen L. (1998) Effects of epinephrine and phenylephrine on QT interval dispersion in congenital long QT syndrome. *J Am Coll Cardiol.* 31: 1400-1405.

[101] Swedberg K, Eneroth P, Kjekshus J, & Wilhelmsen L. (1990) Hormones regulating cardiovascular function in patients with severe congestive heart failure and their relation to mortality. CONSENSUS Trial Study Group. *Circulation.* 82: 1730-1736.

[102] Teitelman G, Baker H, Joh TH, & Reis DJ. (1979) Appearance of catecholamine-synthesizing enzymes during development of rat sympathetic nervous system: possible role of tissue environment. *Proc Natl Acad Sci U S A.* 76: 509-513.

[103] Tidgren B, Hjemdahl P, Theodorsson E, & Nussberger J. (1991) Renal neurohormonal and vascular responses to dynamic exercise in humans. *J Appl Physiol.* 70: 2279-2286.

[104] Torda T, Culman J, & Petriková M. (1987) Distribution of phenylethanolamine-N-methyltransferase in the rat heart: effect of 6-hydroxydopamine. *Eur J Pharmacol.* 141: 305-308.

[105] Tovar OH, Bransford PP, & Jones JL. (1998) Probability of induction and stabilization of ventricular fibrillation with epinephrine. *J Mol Cell Cardiol.* 30: 373-382.

[106] Tovar OH, & Jones JL. (1997) Epinephrine facilitates cardiac fibrillation by shortening action potential refractoriness. *J Mol Cell Cardiol.* 29: 1447-1455.

[107] Trippodo NC. (1981) Total circulatory capacity in the rat. Effects of epinephrine and vasopressin on compliance and unstressed volume. *Circ Res.* 49: 923-931.

[108] van Veldhuisen DJ, Boomsma F, de Kam PJ, Man in't Veld AJ, Crijns HJ, Hampton JR, & Lie KI. (1998) Influence of age on neurohormonal activation and prognosis in patients with chronic heart failure. *Eur Heart J.* 19: 753-760.

[109] Verrier RL. (1990) Behavioral stress, myocardial ischemia, and arrhythmias. In: Zipes DP, Jalife J (eds). *Cardiac Electrophysiology from Cell to Bedside.* Philadelphia, PA: WB Saunders Company, 343-352.

[110] Von Euler US. (1951) Hormones of the sympathetic nervous system and the adrenal medulla. *Br Med J.* 1: 105-108.

[111] Von Euler U, Ikkos D, & Luft R. (1961) Adrenaline excretion during resting conditions and after insulin in adrenalectomized human subjects. *Acta Endocrinol (Copenh).* 38: 441-448.

[112] Ware WA, Lund DD, Subieta AR, & Schmid PG. (1990) Sympathetic activation in dogs with congestive heart failure caused by chronic mitral valve disease and dilated cardiomyopathy. *J Am Vet Med Assoc.* 197: 1475-1481.

[113] Yamada S, Urayama A, Kimura R, Watanabe H, & Ohashi K. (2000) Ameliorating effects of amlodipine on plasma and myocardial catecholamines in BIO 53.58 Syrian hamsters, a model of dilated cardiomyopathy. *Lif Sci.* 67: 3051-3059.

[114] Yeh TC, Vassalle M, & Lin CI. (1992) Arrhythmogenic mechanisms in human atrial and ventricular muscle fibers. *Cardiology.* 80: 205-214.

[115] Zhang Y, Weaver L Jr, Ibeawuchi A, & Olson KR. (1998) Catecholaminergic regulation of venous function in the rainbow trout. *Am J Physiol.* 274: R1195-R1202.

[116] Ziegler MG, Bao X, Kennedy BP, Joyner A, & Enns R. (2002) Location, Development, Control, and Function of Extraadrenal Phenylethanolamine N-Methyltransferase. *Amm N Y Acad Sci.* 971: 76-82.

In: Research Progress on Epinephrine
Editors: A. G. Lawson and R. I. Gorman, pp. 59-71
ISBN: 978-1-60456-443-3

Chapter III

Epinephrine and its Potential Novel Usage in Surgery

Ercan Karacaoglu[1,*], Richard J. Zienowicz[2]
[1]Yeditepe University, School of Medicine, Department of Plastic Surgery, Istanbul, Turkey
[2]Brown University, School of Medicine, Div of Plastic Surgery, Providence, Rhode Island, USA

Abstract

Epinephrine is a natural catecholamine. It is a potent stimulator of both α - and β-adrenergic receptors. Its expression of action might be local that acts in the field of body administered or systematic while administered via one of the intravenous or parenteral routes. The expression of action for epinephrine administered systematically depends on the part of the body and type of adrenergic receptors involved. With its α-1 adrenergic properties on skin and subcutaneous tissue, epinephrine is an extremely potent vasoconstrictor.

Epinephrine, being a potent vasoconstrictor, is used ubiquitously in plastic surgery where concentrations as low as 1:200,000 to 1:400,000 provide sufficient vasoconstriction to decrease bleeding at the operative field.

Recent studies described a sustained epinephrine release model in vivo. Using microspheres, which is a part of a drug delivery system, a sustained epinephrine release is achieved. These studies have shown that sustained epinephrine release caused a vascular augmentation in vivo. This augmentation resulted in favorable morphometric, like increase in vessel wall diameter, number of vessels and dilatation, and hemodynamic alterations.

The data extracted from the studies bodes great potential in surgery. Sustained epinephrine release might be applied in bleeding control of operative fields that lasts

* Mail correspondence to: Ercan Karacaoglu, MD. Atasehir Bulvari Manolya 3-2 Daire 8 Atasehir, Istanbul, 34 758 Turkey. E mail: drercanka@yahoo.com; Phone +90 532 58132 38.

more than a few hours such as in burn surgeries or highly vascularized operative fields such as scalp and face. On the other hand the ability of intentionally augmenting the vascular network in vivo without surgery holds great potential for flap surgery. As a final, it is shown that high epinephrine applied to a soft tissue is causing tissue necrosis. High concentrations of epinephrine release via the aforementioned drug delivery system might be applied to decrease a tumor volume by causing tissue necrosis. In this case, high concentrations of epinephrine would be applied locally and functioning as a 'chemical killer' for tumor cells.

Introduction

Epinephrine is used extensively in daily clinical practice. It is well known and studied that epinephrine has its major effect on vasculature where it plays a significant hemostatic role [1-6]. Although it is clinically used extensively, the data regarding the long term effects of epinephrine on soft tissues is limited [7, 8].

Recent data pertaining long-term local administration of epinephrine to soft tissues have yielded promising results [7-9]. These studies have demonstrated that epinephrine administered by protracted depot time-release technology caused favorable histologic increases in vessel wall diameter and the number of vessels [7, 8]. Finally a more recent data revealed that it is epinephrine that triggers a hypoxia-neovascularization "cascade" and that sustained epinephrine release causes a vascular augmentation in vivo [9].

Epinephrine

Epinephrine is a prototype of direct acting sympathomimetic drugs as it activates all known subtypes of sympathetic nervous system receptors [10].

The sympathetic nervous system is an important regulator of the activities of organs such as heart and peripheral vasculature. The effects of sympathetic stimulation are mediated by release of norepinephrine from nerve terminals and by release of epinephrine from the adrenal medulla epinephrine is transported in the blood to target tissues-in other words epinephrine acts as a hormone. Drugs that mimic the actions of epinephrine or norepinephrine are called sympathomimetic drugs.

Sympathomimetic drugs can be grouped by made of action and by spectrum of receptors that they affect. Drugs such as epinephrine act by a direct mode i.e. they directly interact with and activate adrenoreceptors. A second group of sympathomimetics act indirectly that their actions are dependent on the release of endogenous catecholamine. A third group of sympathomimetics have both direct and indirect actions [11].

Epinephrine Mode of Action and Adrenoreceptors

Molecular mechanism by which catecholamine act has been worked almost a century ago. It is hypothesized that drugs have their effects by interacting with specific receptors.

These receptors are termed as α and β. α receptors are those that exhibit the potency series epinephrine >>norepinephrine >>isoproteronol. β receptors have the potency series isoproterenol >>epinephrine >>norepinephrine. There are at least three subtypes for each of α and β receptors, namely, α_{1A}, α_{1B}, α_{1D}, α_{2A}, α_{2B}, α_{2C} and β_1, β_2, β_3 receptors. β_1 and β_2 receptors are operationally defined by their affinities for epinephrine and norepinephrine. β_1 receptors have approximately equal affinity for epinephrine and norepinephrine, where as β_2 receptors have a higher affinity for epinephrine than for norepinephrine [11, 12].

It is known that there are two major groups of α receptors: α_1 and α_2. The data of subtypes within the α_1 group emerged out of pharmacologic experiments. These experiments indicated complex shapes of agonist dose-response curves of smooth muscle contraction in some tissues as well as differences in antagonist affinities in certain contractile responses. These studies revealed two subtypes of α receptor and a third α receptor subtype has been identified by molecular cloning techniques. These receptors are termed α_{1A}, α_{1B}, α_{1D} receptors. In addition, variants and low affinity subtypes for α receptors are also defined. Clarifying the specific roles and the importance of each of these various subtypes for mediating α_1 receptor response in a variety of organs has been a major area of investigation. Similarly radioligand binding assays, pharmalologic experiments and molecular cloning have identified three α_3 receptor proteins that are products of distinct genes [10, 11].

To complete the section of adrenoreceptors it is worthy to mention about the dopamine receptors. There are five subtypes of dopamine receptors: D_1, D_2, D_3, D_4, and D_5. Further analysis of these receptors is beyond the scope of this chapter.

One of the major features of adrenoreceptors is its *selectivity*. Selectivity reflects preference and it means that a drug may preferentially bind to one subgroup of receptors at concentrations too low to interact with another subgroup. Selectivity is not usually absolute. Higher concentrations related classes of receptor may also interact with the drug [12].

Comparative Ultrastructural Mechanism of Epinephrine

Cells have their own receptors on their surfaces. Adrenergic actions are mediated by these cell surface receptors. These surface receptors are coupled by G proteins to the various effect or proteins whose activities are regulated by those receptors. G proteins of particular importance for adrenoceptor function include G_5, the stimulatory G protein of adenyl cyclase; Gi, the inhibitory G protein of adenyl cyclase; Gq, the protein coupling α receptors to phospholipase C.

Molecular mechanism of α receptors is not clearly defined as of β-receptors. α_1-receptor activation leads to influx of calcium across the membrane in some smooth muscle cells. Where as this activation in many other cells lead to breakdown of polyphosphoinositides into inositol triphosphate and diacylglycerol.

α_1-receptor also activates signal transduction pathways that have traditionally been associated with peptide growth factors. α_1-receptors have been found to activate mitogen activated kinases (MAP kinases) and polyphosphoinositol3-kinase (PI-3-kinase). It is believed that these findings might be related to the α 1-receptor-mediated stimulation of cell growth.

Contrary to fact, the mechanism of action of β -adrenergic has been studied in detail. Activation of β subtypes results in activation of adenyl cyclase and increased conversion of ATP to cAMP. cAMP is the major second messenger of β -receptor activation. β -agonists may activate voltage-sensitive calcium channels in the heart.

Responses after stimulation of adrenoceptors are variable and dynamic. This is known as receptor regulation. After a tissue has been exposed for a certain period of time to an agonist, that tissue often becomes less responsive to further stimulation by the same agent. This phenomenon is known as *desensitization.* This process has potential clinical significance as it might restrict the response to the certain adrenergic agents. Desensitization might occur even within minutes [12].

Organ System Effects of Epinephrine

Epinephrine is a potent stimulator of both α and β adrenergic receptors. Its effects on target organs are complex. In this chapter epinephrine effects on only cardiovascular system and related miscellaneous organs will be discussed.

1. Effects on Cardiovascular System

a. *Blood vessels:* The skin vessels have predominantly α receptors. These vessels constrict in the presence of epinephrine. Epinephrine has the same effect on the splanchnic vessels. But vessels in skeletal muscle may constrict or dilate depending on whether α and β receptors are activated. The chief vascular action of epinephrine is exerted on the smaller arterioles and precapillary sphincters, although veins and large arteries also respond to the agent. Epinephrine with its vasoconstrictor effect markedly reduces cutaneous blood flow, constricting precapillary vessels and subcapillary venules. This cutaneous vasoconstriction accounts for a marked decrease in blood flow in the hands and feet. The post injection congestion of mucosa following injection of epinephrine is probably due to changes in vascular reactivity as a result of tissue hypoxia rather than to β -receptor stimulation of drug on mucosal vessels. Therapeutic doses of epinephrine increases blood flow to skeletal muscles. This is due in part to a powerful β_2-receptor vasodilator action. If a α-blocker agent is given, the vasodilatation in muscle is more pronounced, the total peripheral resistance is decreased and the mean blood pressure falls. This is known as epinephrine reversal.
b. *Cardiac effects:* Epinephrine is known and widely used as a powerful cardiac stimulant. Epinephrine acts directly on the predominant β_1-receptors of the myocardium and of the cells of the pacemakers and conducting tissues; β_2 and α receptors are also available in the heart.
c. *Other organ system vasculature*: The effect of epinephrine on cerebral circulation is indirect and related to systemic blood pressure. Intravenous infusion of 0.1 microgram/kg/min markedly increases hepatic blood flow and decreases splanchnic vascular resistance and reduces renal blood flow by as much as 40%. Arterial and

venous pulmonary pressures are raised. Coronary blood flow is enhanced by epinephrine or by cardiac sympathetic stimulation [10-12].

2. Miscellaneous Effects

Epinephrine reduces circulating plasma volume by loss of protein-free fluid to the extra cellular space, thereby increasing erythrocyte and plasma protein concentrations. These effects are mainly exists under nonphysiologic conditions i.e. shock, hemorrhage, hypotension and anesthesia. Epinephrine increases total leukocyte count but causes eosinopenia. Epinephrine accelerates blood coagulation on effect probably due to increased activity of factor V. Sweating and pilomotor activity are seen after intradermal injection of very dilute solutions but these effects are not seen after systemic administration. Although epinephrine does not directly excite skeletal muscle, if facilitates neuromuscular transmission, particularly that following prolonged rapid stimulation of the motor nerve. This effect appears to involve both α and β receptors. Stimulation of adrenergic receptors causes a more rapid increase in transmitter release from the somatic motoneuron. Epinephrine produces a transient rise in the concentration of K^+ in plasma, mainly due to release of the ion from the liver. This hyperkalemia is followed by a more prolonged fall in plasma K^+. During these changes hepatic K^+ rapidly enters the blood and is taken up by muscle. Subsequently the pool of K^+in muscle falls during the period of hypokalemia and is transferred to the liver [10,11,12].

Large or repeated doses of epinephrine given to experimental animals lead to damage to arterial walls and myocardium so severe as to cause the appearance of necrotic areas, indistinguishable in the heart from myocardial infarcts. Similar lesions occur in many patients with pheochromocytoma [11].

Epinephrine's Current Usage in Surgery

Reduction of regional blood flow is desirable for achieving hemostasis in surgery, for reducing diffusion of local anesthetics away from the site of administration, and for reducing mucous membrane congestion. In each instance α receptor activation is desired, and the choice of agent depends upon the maximal efficacy required, the desired duration of action, and the route of administration. Effective pharmacologic hemostasis, often necessary for facial, oral and nasopharyngeal surgery, requires drugs of high efficacy that can be administered in high concentration by local application.

Nasal and Sinus Surgery

Epinephrine is usually applied topically in nasal packs mostly for septal, sinus and concha surgery. While are they so effective? The vascular bed in nasal mucosa is highly vascularized and an extensive sinusoidal network of large capacitance vessel is present deep within the submucosa. When this network of venous sinusoids is engorged with blood, swollen mucosa reduces the size of the airway lumen and congestion ensues. Nasal vasculature tone is strongly influenced by the sympathetic agonists and the only drugs approved specifically to relieve vascular nasal obstruction are alpha agonist agents. Due to their vasoconstrictor action epinephrine oppose vasodilatation, reducing nasal airway resistance and thus facilitating nose breathing.

Local anesthetics with epinephrine combinations are often used to reduce bleeding and hence improve the operating field in septal, sinus and conchal surgery. [13, 14, 15]. It is one of the most used combinations for epistaxis. It is well known that cocaine is a potent vasoconstrictor. Recent reports compare cocaine flakes with local anesthetics with epinephrine and concluded that the solution of local anesthetic and epinephrine is an effective and safe anesthetic for patients undergoing surgery under local anesthesia [14].

Miscellaneous

Application of epinephrine in current surgery and surgical procedures is not limited to the nasal and sinus surgery. It is also used in nasopharynx, oropharynx, palatal, oral surgery including gingival string for gingivectomy and adenoidectomy [16]. Occasionally, cocaine is mixed with epinephrine for maximum hemostasis and local anesthesia in any of these procedures. Epinephrine is also used as a routine agent in periodontal surgery and endodonthic therapy [17, 18, 19].

It is a well established practice to apply epinephrine during *burn surgery*. It is always a question of debate how reliable is the epinephrine if it has to be used for patient with a large area of burn surface. A recent study investigated this reliability and prospectively studied the acute cardiovascular responses to epinephrine administered subcutaneously and topically during burn surgery. The increase in mean arterial pressure was not clinically found significant, did not require intervention, and did not appear to be related to the type of wound that received epinephrine (donor site vs. burn wound), or the depth of anesthesia, analgesia, or sedation. On the basis of these findings, the use of subcutaneous and topical epinephrine appears to be safe and produces minimal acute cardiovascular effects [20].

Epinephrine use in certain area of body is a question of reliability. This is due to the belief of possible vascular compromising end results of epinephrine. Little attention has been paid to analyze the evidence that created this belief to see whether it is valid. The significance is that elective epinephrine *finger* injection has been shown to remove the need for a tourniquet, and therefore delete sedation and general anesthesia for much of hand surgery. The evidence that created the dogma that epinephrine should not be injected into the fingers is clearly not valid. However, there is considerable valid evidence in the literature that supports the tenet that properly used epinephrine in the fingers is safe, and that it removes the need for a tourniquet and therefore removes the need for sedation and general anesthesia for many hand operations [21].

A recent report compared the cellular and ultrastructural changes in the urethral wall following application of different hemostasis techniques in a rabbit model of *hypospadias surgery*. They concluded that hemostasis techniques applied for maintaining a bloodless surgical field during hypospadias repair may lead to ischemia/reperfusion tissue damage in the urethral wall and suggested that epinephrine injection might have resulted in more prominent cellular changes compared to tourniquet techniques and advised for further experimental and human studies to draw a firm conclusion [22].

Endoscopic treatment of ulcer bleeding with epinephrine is an also a well established mode of treatment. Upper gastrointestinal bleeding secondary to ulcer disease occurs commonly and results in significant patient morbidity. Carefully performed endoscope provides an accurate diagnosis of the source of the upper gastrointestinal bleeding hemorrhage and can reliably identify those high-risk subgroups that may benefit most from endoscopic hemostasis. Epinephrine injection and either thermal coaptive coagulation- with multipolar or heater probe- or endoclips is the gold standard. Effective endoscopic hemostasis with epinephrine of ulcer bleeding is shown significantly improve outcomes by reducing rebleeding, transfusion requirement, and need for surgery, as well as reduce cost of medical care [23, 24, 25].

Epinephrine *in regional blocks* are also very well known mode of application in surgery. Combining α agonists with some local anesthetics greatly prolongs the duration of infiltration nerve block; the total dose of local anesthetic and the probability of toxicity can therefore be reduced. Epinephrine, 1:200,000 is the favored agent for this application. Recently, epinephrine-augmented hypotensive epidural anesthesia is also found to be an effective method to avoid the use of a tourniquet during total knee arthroplasty without the negative effects on perioperative hemoglobin values [26].

Potential Novel Usage of Epinephrine in Surgery

All aforementioned studies bodes great potential in epinephrine applications. Some of these techniques are novel. Without exception, all of these applications consist of single shot application of epinephrine. In other words none of them are related to the long term effects of epinephrine on the field that is applied nor there a sustained application of epinephrine on these field of treatment or surgery.

More recent studies aimed to focus on long term effects of epinephrine on soft tissue it applied [7, 8, 9]. The objectives of these studies are as follows:

1. to investigate the effect of long term local release of epinephrine from a drug delivery system on rat abdominal skin vasculature which most likely contains alpha adrenoreceptors and to evaluate the pharmacodynamic and pharmacokinetic properties of drug delivery system.
2. to determine whether epinephrine can induce a hypoxia-neovascularization cascade to trigger vascular proliferation within soft tissues.
3. to increase flap tolerance to the critical period of vasospasm that occurs after flap elevation,

In reconstructive surgery, flap reconstruction is maybe the most frequently performed procedures. It is true for flap surgeries in plastic and reconstructive surgery and in other surgeries that use flap in any part of their surgical procedures i.e. general surgery, urology, cardiothoracic surgery, orthopedic surgery.

Despite new flap designs and surgical technique, ischemic necrosis is still a substantial complication of all types flap surgery. [27, 28] Numerous studies were advocated to improve the viability of flap surgery or subside necrosis in flaps elevated. Nevertheless, the surgical delay procedure is the only proven technique that can extend reliably the area of flap viability than can be achieved by a single-stage operation. This is essential for both clinical and experimental procedures [41]. In clinical practice, a surgical delay is performed to increase the survival area of a random-pattern flap, to improve circulation to an axial flap, to combat the insult of a twist when the flap is transferred, or to increase the survival of the random adjacent tissue of an axial-pattern flap by the strategic ligation of vessels along the flap axis at time intervals. These measurements are almost mandatory especially for certain type of surgeries i.e. reconstruction after a cancer surgery [30, 31, 32, 33] Despite many advances in flap surgery and our greater understanding of flap behavior, no unifying theory on the mechanism of the delay process explains this surgical phenomenon adequately [29]. Numerous studies have shown that arterial flow has been shown to improve and reorient during delay [34, 35]. It is also shown that flap edema reduces, presumably because of improved, venous and lymphatic drainage, and this is also shown to be an effect of the delay process [36].

A recent study postulated that the mechanism promoting the delay phenomenon is the dilatation of choke anastomotic vessels and their related vascular tributaries [8]. It is well known that flaps undergo metabolic chaos after flap elevation. Preparing flaps by artificial stress, before elevation, appears to confer resistance to these deleterious effects. In this study, the improvement of flap survival with the chemical delay technique proved markedly similar to the improvement of survival with standard surgical delay. Speculations made on the mechanism of this phenomenon. It could be the active dilatation of the choke vessels beyond simple relaxation of sympathetic tone of the smooth muscle wall. But two factors are considered to be the mechanism of delay: the physical effect of blood and hypoxia [9] where the postulated mechanism is considered to be primarily related to a dynamic vascular response rather than to persistent, prolonged hypoxia.

There is no doubt that hypoxia is a potent stimulus for neovascularization [6, 17] but molecular mechanism to how hypoxia triggers neovascularization is still unclear. Investigations of the physical, chemical, and physiological events include work on vascular endothelium-derived relaxing factors, free radicals, nitric oxide, shear stress, hem oxygenase-1 [37, 38, 39, 40].

Dhar and Taylor's rabbit flap experiment illustrated graphically the anatomic effect of hypoxia on the caliber of the vessels connecting across the scar perimeter of the flap [29]. They demonstrated that if the perimeter of the flap is followed proximally to distally, the caliber of the arteries connecting the flap to its base increases as the flap becomes more hypoxic. Based on these findings the recent study is developed and injection of epinephrine microspheres into the flap is used to mimic hypoxic background of ischemia after flap elevation [7]. In this study epinephrine is used to ensure continuous vasoconstriction by the direct effect of epinephrine on receptors of skin, which is known to be a potent stimulus for neovascularization [8]. It is postulated that this vasoconstrictive event has its major effect on the choke anastomotic vessel wall. A sustained drug delivery system for epinephrine is defined and studied in a different paper [7]. It is shown that elution properties that allow delivery of epinephrine for approximately 7 days appears sufficient to promote permanent anatomic changes to the vessel walls. And this finding is correlated with the observation Dhar and Taylor that a 7-day period after surgical delay is adequate if not optimal for achievement of the salubrious vasculometabolic effects [7, 8, 29].

It will be worthy to describe how this sustained drug delivery system works. The system is designed as an experimental model to deliver epinephrine to discrete area of local soft tissues for a limited time. This system has two components one is microspheres and the other one is active agent to be delivered where it is epinephrine in the study. Microspheres are fine spherical porous particles with a diameter of 3-10 micron. They are biodegradable. Investigators in the field of medicinal chemistry, pharmaceutics and tissue engineering uses biodegradable microspheres as a component of the long term controlled release of a variety of pharmacological agents in the last two decades [41, 42]. Microspheres serve as a vehicle for drug transport and delivery. The advantage of the microspehere drug delivery system loaded with epinephrine is the ability to deliver active agent for a long duration, with the effects ideally limited to a local region. Duration of release of the active agent is also possible to determine by this system. This has an advantage of avoiding possible systemic side effects of the agent delivered. This advantage is extremely important for agents that could have an extreme effect profile on body systems such as epinephrine and hormones. And this procedure does not require multiple surgical procedures but one [7].

As a conclusion the study demonstrated that the method of chemical delay bears an uncanny resemblance to conventional surgical delay both in vascular anatomic alterations and inevitably in surgical outcome. That epinephrine administered by sustained drug delivery system release technology causes favorable hemodynamic alterations to the local tissue milieu is certain. It is shown that adrenergic agonist effect of epinephrine is the seminal event initiating the delay cascade [9].

Clinical extrapolation of these experiments to flap surgery is straightforward [7, 8, 9].

Briefly this novel use of epinephrine ensures two different advantages: sustained vasoconstriction and vascular augmentation. Both of them could be combined in clinical practice. Or these two features could be postulated separately.

1. *Sustained Vasoconstriction:* Sustained epinephrine release is shown to cause a continuous vasoconstriction. This vasoconstriction causes decreased blood flow within the first three days after epinephrine application [9] where the dosage and duration of release is reported to be adjustable. Adjustability of the sustained epinephrine release is one of the superiority of the system. By this feature a sustained vasoconstriction from three days to a few hours is possible to adjust. Hemostasis is known as one of the principles of surgery since and before Halsted. Bloodless field of surgery is not only for to make surgical procedure precise but also for lowering complications. This is especially true for the surgical fields that have a rich vascular network. These include the following procedures: head and neck cancer surgery, head and neck reconstruction, scalp surgery , nasal surgery, maxillofacial trauma, orthognathic surgery, periorbital surgery, facial cosmetic surgery (including forehead lifting, blepheroplasty, midface lifting, face lifting, neck lifting, modifications of

face lifting such as deep plane lifting, MACS, SMAS lifting, malar augmentation, chin augmentation etc.) .

Another area of application is surgical field that has a predilection to bleeding. These include the followings: majority of oncologic surgeries (head and neck, skin, melanoma, mediastine, bowel, deep pelvic surgeries including prostate), fresh burn surgery, burn deformity surgeries, flap surgeries, graft surgeries, recently operated surgical fields etc.

Dosage of epinephrine to be delivered is also key that a higher dosage may cause a necrosis instead of hemostasis within the tissues applied [9]. Necrosis of arterial wall and myocardium has been reported in many patients with pheochromocytoma [11]. These two studies imply the role of large doses of epinephrine in vivo. This might bode great potential in oncologic surgery. It is well known that cytoreductive surgery is one of the procedures that serves as a relief for numerous conditions i.e. tumor with an unresectable anatomic location, a tumor which is adjacent to the vital anatomic structures or a tumor with enormous dimensions where a surgical approach such as a resection may not give a satisfactory result as an initial procedure. In these circumstances an epinephrine loaded drug delivery system applied to the center of the tumor may diminish the dimension of the mass. This would be debulking feature of this system. Henceforth, large and sustained doses of epinephrine might act as a 'chemical killer'. Ongoing studies on this issue seem promising.

2. *Vascular Augmentation:* This augmentation consists of favorable increase in vessel wall diameter, number of vessels. A vascular dilatation accompanies with these ultrastructural changes. It is also shown that a hemodynamic alteration also exists. This bodes great potential in reconstructive surgery and in surgeries using flaps or grafts. Augmenting the vascularity of certain flaps before elevation should result in an increase in the survival of those flaps. This will decrease the possibility of flap necrosis and untoward complications of flap surgeries. Injection of epinephrine drug delivery system as an office procedure only 12 days before definitive surgery might have a potential effect to reduce flap necrosis. This is definitely would be very cost effective and would increase the success of surgery.

   Similarly, augmenting the vascular network will ensure a higher ratio of graft take for certain poorly vascularized recipient areas. Chronic ulcers with poor and ill vascularization have a limited wound healing potential. Grafting as the simplest method of reconstruction is theorically ideal but practically frustrating. Application of epinephrine loaded drug delivery system for a certain time before grafting might give promising results. It might also have a potential effect on fat graft survival. Fat tissue resorption after grafting is a constant problem of this procedure. Numerous attempts had been made to increase graft take and decrease fat tissue resorption. Nevertheless a 30-80 % resorption rate is anticipated. Injection of epinephrine loaded drug delivery system well before fat grafting might also increase fat tissue take. Similarly, augmenting the vascularity of recipient tissues might also increase the take of composite grafts.

References

[1] Brantner JN, Peterson HD. The role of vasoconstrictors in control of blood loss in reduction mammaplasty. *Plast Reconstr Surg.* 1985 Mar; 75(3):339-41.

[2] Solomon MP. Tumescent technique as an adjunct to breast implant removal and capsulectomy. *Ann Plast Surg.* 2000 May; 44(5):495-7.

[3] Brezel BS, McGeever KE, Stein JM. Epinephrine v thrombin for split-thickness donor site hemostasis.*J Burn Care Rehabil.* 1987 Mar-Apr;8(2):132-4.

[4] Karaoglu S, Dogru K, Kabak S, Inan M, Halici M. Effects of epinephrine in local anesthetic mixtures on hemodynamics and view quality during knee arthroscopy. *Knee Surg Sports Traumatol Arthrosc.* 2002 Jul; 10(4):226-8.

[5] Rowlands RG, Hicklin L, Hinton AE. Novel use of nebulised adrenaline in the treatment of secondary oropharyngeal haemorrhage.*J Laryngol Otol.* 2002 Feb;116(2):123-4.

[6] Wilhelm BJ, Blackwell SJ, Miller JH, Mancoll JS, Dardano T, Tran A, Phillips LG. Do not use epinephrine in digital blocks: myth or truth? *Plast Reconstr Surg.* 2001 Feb; 107(2):393-7.

[7] Karacaoglu E, Cermik H, Yurdun T, Zienowicz RJ. Effect of long-term application of epinephrine on rat skin vasculature. Experimental study. *Microsurgery* 2002, 22:288-294.

[8] Karacaoglu E, Yuksel F, Turan SO, Zienowicz RJ. Chemical delay: An Alternative to surgical delay: Experimental study. *Ann Plast Surg* 2002, 49:73-81.

[9] Karacaoglu E, Bayram I, Celikoz B, Zienowicz RJ. Does sustained epinephrine release trigger a hypoxia-neovascularization cascade? *Plast Reconstr Surg. 2007,119:85.*

[10] Hoffman BB. Adrenoreceptor-activating and other sympathomimetic drugs. In: Katzung BG (Ed.). *Basic and Clinical Pharmacology.* 8th Ed. New York: McGraw-Hill, 2001, Pp 120-127.

[11] Moore KE. Drugs affecting the sympathetic nervous system. In: Brody TM, Larner J, Minneman KP (Eds.). *Human Pharmacology, Molecular to Clinical.* St Louis: Mosby-Year Boo, 1998, Pp 119-132.

[12] Weiner N. Norepinephrine, epinephrine and the sympathomimetic amines. In: Gilman AG, Goodman LS, Murad F (Eds.). *The Pharmacological Basis of Therapeutics.* New York: MacMillan; 1985, Pp 145-180.

[13] McClymont LG, Crowther JA. Local anaesthetic with vasoconstrictor combinations in septal surgery. *J Laryngol Otol.* 1988 Sep; 102(9):793-5.

[14] Bizakis JG, Lachanas VA, Drivas EI, Kyrmizakis DE, Prokopakis EP, Benakis AA, Helidonis ES. Cocaine flakes versus tetracaine/adrenaline solution for local anaesthesia in septoplasty. *Rhinology.* 2004 Dec; 42(4):236-8.

[15] Corboz MR, Rivelli MA, Mingo GG, McLeod RL, Varty L, Jia Y, Hey JA. Mechanism of decongestant activity of alpha(2)-adrenoceptor agonists.*Pulm Pharmacol Ther.* 2007 Jul 17 [Epub ahead of print].

[16] Huins CT, Narula AA. Topical adrenaline in control of intraoperative bleeding in adenoidectomy: a randomised control trial. *Clin Otolaryngol.* 2007 Apr;32(2):136.

[17] Cohen HP, Cha BY, Spångberg LS. Endodontic anesthesia in mandibular molars: a clinical study. *J Endod.* 1993 Jul; 19(7):370-3.

[18] Moore PA, Doll B, Delie RA, Hersh EV, Korostoff J, Johnson S, Goodson JM, Halem S, Palys M, Leonel JS, Kozlowski VA, Peterson C, Hutcheson M. Hemostatic and anesthetic efficacy of 4% articaine HCl with 1:200,000 epinephrine and 4% articaine HCl with 1:100,000 epinephrine when administered intraorally for periodontal surgery. *J Periodontol.* 2007 Feb; 78(2):247-53.

[19] Davenport RE, Porcelli RJ, Iacono VJ, Bonura CF, Mallis GI, Baer PN. Effects of anesthetics containing epinephrine on catecholamine levels during periodontal surgery. *J Periodontol.* 1990 Sep;61(9):553-8.

[20] Cartotto R, Kadikar N, Musgrave MA, Gomez M, Cooper AB. What are the acute cardiovascular effects of subcutaneous and topical epinephrine for hemostasis during burn surgery? *J Burn Care Rehabil.* 2003 Sep-Oct; 24(5):297-305.

[21] Thomson CJ, Lalonde DH, Denkler KA, Feicht AJ. A critical look at the evidence for and against elective epinephrine use in the finger. *Plast Reconstr Surg.* 2007 Jan;119 (1):260-6.

[22] Kajbafzadeh AM, Payabvash S, Tavangar SM, Salmasi AH, Sadeghi Z, Elmi A, Tirgari F, Razavi AE. Comparison of different techniques for hemostasis in a rabbit model of hypospadias repair. *J Urol.* 2007 Dec; 178(6):2555-60.

[23] Katsinelos P, Kountouras J, Chatzimavroudis G, Zavos C, Paroutoglou G, Pilpilidis I, Papaziogas B. A novel technique of injection treatment for endoscopic sphincterotomy-induced hemorrhage. *Endoscopy.* 2007 Jul; 39(7):631-6.

[24] Kovacs TO, Jensen DM. Endoscopic treatment of ulcer bleeding. *Curr Treat Options Gastroenterol.* 2007 Mar; 10(2):143-8.

[25] Hsu PI, Lai KH, Lo GH. Is epinephrine the best solution for large-volume endoscopic injection of peptic ulcer bleeding? *Gastrointest Endosc.* 2005 Jul; 62(1):195.

[26] Kiss H, Raffl M, Neumann D, Hutter J, Dorn U. Epinephrine-augmented hypotensive epidural anesthesia replaces tourniquet use in total knee replacement. *Clin Orthop Relat Res.* 2005 Jul; (436):184-9.

[27] Dang CM, Forrest CR, Morris S. Pharmacological augmentation of skin flap viability: a hypothesis to mimic the surgical delay phenomenon or a wishful thought. *Ann Plast Surg* 1989; 22:293–306.

[28] Daniel RK, Kerrigan CL. Principles and physiology of skin flap surgery. In: *McCarthy JG, ed. Plastic surgery.* Vol. 1.Philadelphia: WB Saunders, 1990:275–328.

[29] Dhar SC, Taylor IG. The delay phenomenon: the story unfolds. *Plast Reconstr Surg* 1999;104:2079–2091.

[30] Pinsolle V, Grinfeder C, Mathoulin-Pelissier S, Faucher A.Complications analysis of 266 immediate breast reconstructions.*J Plast Reconstr Aesthet Surg.* 2006; 59(10): 1017-24.

[31] Salhab M, Al Sarakbi W, Joseph A, Sheards S, Travers J, Mokbel K. Skin-sparing mastectomy and immediate breast reconstruction: patient satisfaction and clinical outcome. *J Clin Oncol.* 2006 Feb;11(1):51-4.

[32] Gabbay JS, Eby JB, Kulber DA.The midabdominal TRAM flap for breast reconstruction in morbidly obese patients. *Plast Reconstr Surg. 2005 Mar;*115(3):764-70.

[33] Kronowitz SJ, Hunt KK, Kuerer HM, Babiera G, McNeese MD, Buchholz TA, Strom EA, Robb GL. Delayed-immediate breast reconstruction. *Plast Reconstr Surg.* 2004 May;113(6):1617-28.

[34] Sunuki S, Isshiki N, Ohtsuka M, et al. Experimental study on "delay" phenomenon in relation to flap width and ischemia. *Br J Plast Surg* 1988; 41:389–392.

[35] Garcia PB, Nieto CS, Ortega JMR. Morphological changes in the vascularization of delayed flaps in rabbits. *Br J Plast Surg* 1991; 44:285–288.

[36] Angel MF, Ramasastry SS, Swartz WM, et al. The critical relationship between free radicals and degrees of ischemia: evidence for tissue intolerance of marginal perfusion. *Plast Reconstr Surg* 1988; 81:223–227.

[37] Bevan JA. Shear stress, the endothelium and the balance between flow induced contraction and dilatation in animals and man. *Int J Microcirc Clin Exp* 1997;17:248–251.

[38] Shu MG, Guo XT, Zhen HN, Han Y, Chen FL, Li LW, Guo SZ. Enhancing skin flap survival by a cell-permeable wild-type survivin. *Med Hypotheses.* 2007;69(4):888-91.

[39] Kubulus D, Roesken F, Amon M, Rücker M, Bauer M, Bauer I, Menger MD.Mechanism of the delay phenomenon: tissue protection is mediated by heme oxygenase-1.*Am J Physiol Heart Circ Physiol.* 2004 Nov;287(5):H2332-40.

[40] Barker JH, Frank J, Bidiwala SB, Stengel CK, Carroll SM, Carroll CM, van Aalst V, Anderson GL. An animal model to study microcirculatory changes associated with vascular delay.*Br J Plast Surg.* 1999 Mar; 52(2):133-42.

[41] Couvreur P, Puisieux F. Nano and microparticles for the delivery of polypeptides and proteins. *Adv Drug Rev* 1993; 10:141.

[42] Cleek RL, Rege AA, Denner LA, Eskin SG, Mikos AG. Inhibition of smooth muscle cell growth in vitro by antisense oligodeoxynucleotide released from poly (DL-lactic-co-glycolicacid microparticles. *J Biomed Mater Res* 1997 Jun 15; 35(4):525-30.

In: Research Progress on Epinephrine
Editors: A. G. Lawson and R. I. Gorman, pp. 73-94
ISBN: 978-1-60456-443-3

Chapter IV

Platelets and Epinephrine

Andreas C. Eriksson and Per A. Whiss
Division of Drug Research/Pharmacology, Department of Medical and Health Sciences, Linköping University, SE-58183, Linköping, Sweden

Abstract

Epinephrine is one substance among several others that contributes to platelet activation. Platelet activation is crucial for normal haemostasis but can also be deleterious in the setting of thrombosis. The activating effect of epinephrine on platelets is achieved through α_2-adrenergic receptors (α_2-ARs). Present on platelets are also inhibitory β-adrenergic receptors. However, the importance of these latter receptors for *in vivo* platelet function is unknown. Signalling from the α_2-ARs go through the G_z-protein. A result of this is lowered levels of intracellular cAMP but the signalling pathways stimulated by epinephrine are far more complex than this. Consequently, this is a research area that needs more investigation. It is also important to consider activation with epinephrine in the context of other platelet activators, since this is the case *in vivo*. Epinephrine is known to develop synergistic effects with platelet activators such as thrombin, lysophosphatidic acid (LPA), platelet-activating factor (PAF) and serotonin. It has actually been emphasized that epinephrine cannot function on its own on platelets but needs to cooperate with other activators. Furthermore, synergistic platelet adhesion and aggregation induced *in vitro* by epinephrine combined with LPA is dependent on secretion of adenosine-di-phosphate (ADP). Thus, in these cases two additional activators are needed besides epinephrine to achieve platelet activation. The importance of epinephrine for thrombus formation *in vivo* is not totally clear but several studies support a connection between increased levels of epinephrine and cardiovascular events. Increased levels of epinephrine might synergize with other platelet activators released after atherosclerotic plaque rupture resulting in accelerated thrombosis.

Introduction

The physiological role of platelets is to prevent blood loss after vessel injury. In short, platelets first adhere to extracellular proteins such as collagen and von Willebrand factor (vWf), which is followed by adhesion between platelets (aggregation) mediated by fibrinogen [1,2]. Adhesion receptors involved in this process are the glycoprotein (GP)Ib-IX-V and the integrins $\alpha_2\beta_1$ and $\alpha_{IIb}\beta_3$. GPIb-IX-V binds vWf and induces a rolling phenomenon, which reduces the speed of platelet movement. This allows stronger interactions between $\alpha_2\beta_1$ and collagen and between $\alpha_{IIb}\beta_3$ and vWf resulting in firm arrest of the platelets. Finally, binding of fibrinogen to $\alpha_{IIb}\beta_3$ mediates platelet aggregation. However, the process of platelet adhesion and aggregation is far more complicated than this. In order for platelets to attach to a surface they need to get activated. Activation induces the formation of pseudopods, which increases the effective surface area available for adhesion. Furthermore, platelet activation results in conformational changes in the $\alpha_2\beta_1$ and $\alpha_{IIb}\beta_3$-receptors, which are necessary for binding of those receptors to their ligands. The process of platelet activation is very complex involving a lot of different mediators. Initial activating signalling is induced by the surface interactions with vWf, collagen and fibrinogen described above. In addition, platelets are also activated by soluble agonists. The most potent soluble platelet agonist is thrombin, which is produced by the coagulation cascade in the case of vessel injury. Other activators such as adenosine-di-phosphate (ADP) and thromboxane A_2 (TXA_2) are released from platelets following platelet activation. Epinephrine, which is present in plasma, is also able to act as a platelet activator and might as well be released from activated platelets [3,4].

Platelet Adrenergic Receptors

The platelet activating effect of epinephrine have been known since the beginning of the 1960´s [5]. This study also showed that the activating effect of epinephrine was inhibited by the unselective α-adrenergic antagonist phentolamine. Later on, functional studies using platelet aggregometry and different α-adrenergic agonists/antagonists suggested that α-adrenergic receptors (α-ARs) on platelets were of the α_2-subtype [6,7]. Also, the presence of α_2- but not α_1-ARs have been confirmed by pharmacological displacement studies [8]. Through cloning experiments it was shown that the gene for the human platelet α_2-AR is located on chromosome 10 [9]. Further research concerning α_2-ARs has identified three different subtypes and current nomenclature states that the α_2-AR present on platelets is of the α_{2A}-subtype [10]. Platelets also express β-ARs. This is known from early studies showing that the β-agonist isoprenaline inhibited platelet aggregation [11]. The presence of β-ARs on platelets have also been confirmed from experiments using β-antagonists [12] and the β-ARs have been shown to be of the β_2-subtype [13]. It is also known that stimulation of β_2-ARs on platelets result in an increase in intracellular cAMP [13,14]. The presence of both α_2 and β_2-ARs on platelets has stimulated research aimed at investigating the relative contributions of the respective receptors for platelet function. First of all, there is a discrepancy in the amount of α_2 versus β_2-ARs expressed on platelets, with α_2 exceeding β_2 by approximately threefold on human platelets [15]. As will become clear from our discussion, it is signalling through the more numerous α_2-ARs that result in the platelet activating effect exerted by epinephrine. As mentioned above, signalling through β_2-ARs instead have reversed effect resulting in platelet inhibition [11]. The apparent opposite effects exerted by α- and β-AR stimulation respectively is as interesting as it is confusing. It might be suggested that the effect observed in a particular situation is dependent on the concentration of epinephrine. A potentiating effect of 5 nmol/L of epinephrine on ADP-induced platelet activation was dependent on the presence of the β-blocker propranolol [16]. The potentiating effect of 10 nmol/L epinephrine was not affected by propranolol, suggesting that β-AR stimulation is only important at low epinephrine concentrations. These results are further strengthened by the observation that epinephrine at a similar dose (2.73 nmol/L) can activate the platelet inhibiting cGMP-signalling pathway through β-AR stimulation [17]. Contrary to this, platelet activating effects are dependent on high concentrations of epinephrine [18]. Also, epinephrine is in general described as a platelet activator, which makes it important to discuss these results suggesting both activating and inhibiting effects of epinephrine in a physiological context. The basal plasma level of epinephrine is less than 1 nmol/L and it is only moderately elevated in different types of stress [19-21]. This would suggest that epinephrine *in vivo* should act as a platelet inhibitor, contrary to general belief. However, the *in vivo* situation is complicated by the fact that platelets secrete epinephrine [3], which actually contributes to platelet aggregation [4]. It is therefore possible that the epinephrine concentration might be locally elevated in the close vicinity of activated platelets. Also, the *in vivo* situation is extremely complex with several platelet activators being present simultaneously with epinephrine. It is well-known that there is a great deal of cooperation between different platelet activators and this might result in platelet activation induced by relatively low concentrations of epinephrine in the presence of other activators. It is therefore reasonable to assume that local increase in epinephrine concentration induced by secretion as well as potentiation by other activators results in platelet activating effects of epinephrine *in vivo*. The question then remains regarding the physiologic relevance of signalling through β-adrenergic receptors. Most studies performed in healthy volunteers have shown no effect on platelet function of β-blocker administration *in vivo* [18]. The relevance of β-adrenergic signalling *in vivo* is still unsolved and demand further investigation. We speculate that signalling through β-adrenergic receptors by low doses of epinephrine might be important during resting conditions to keep platelets in an unactivated state. Other more potent inhibitors also present at rest, such as PGI_2 and NO released from the endothelium, might mask these effects making these possible effects of epinephrine difficult to observe in experimental settings.

Platelet Activation

Before discussing the details of epinephrine-induced effects on platelets it is important to consider platelet activation in general. The great diversity of platelet activating substances suggests that activation of platelets *in vivo* is extremely complex. Most probably there is interplay between several platelet activators, which lead to final platelet activation. Also, the presence of several platelet activators creates a back-up system where the loss of one activator could be compensated for by another. Consequently, a lot of today's platelet-related research is focused on synergistic effects achieved by combining different activators. The approach to use concerted action of activators have, for example, been suggested to be especially important in pharmacodynamic studies of anti-platelet agents [22,23]. Experiments performed *in vitro* for this purpose are most often performed with the aim of investigating combinations of two or three activators. This is far from the *in vivo* situation concerning the number of activators present, but it is an important step towards the understanding of cross-talk between platelet activators. Many of the soluble platelet agonists act through G-protein-coupled receptors [24]. G-proteins come in many different shapes and subtypes. Especially important for platelet activation are G_q, G_i and $G_{12/13}$. Stimulation of these G-proteins activates different intracellular signalling pathways. G_q activates phospholipase C-β which in turn cleaves phosphatidylinositol-(4,5)-bisphosphate (PIP_2) into diacylglycerol (DAG) and inositol tris-phosphate (IP_3). The consequences of this are elevations of intracellular calcium $[Ca^{2+}]_i$ and activation of protein kinase C (PKC). G_i-proteins in turn act by inhibiting adenylyl cyclase leading to decreased levels of cAMP whereas $G_{12/13}$ activates the small GTPase RhoA, which is involved in reorganization of the actin cytoskeleton. Consequently, stimulation of the different G-proteins result in activation of different signalling pathways that all contribute to platelet activation. The cooperation becomes clear when considering the activating pathways induced by different activators. The thrombin-binding PAR1 and PAR4 receptors as well as the TP-receptor which binds TXA_2 are all coupled to both G_q and G_{13}. ADP in turn utilizes two receptors, P2Y1 and P2Y12, which couple to G_q and G_i respectively. Furthermore, as will be discussed in detail, α_2-ARs are suggested to be coupled to a specific subset of G_i-proteins called G_z.

In light of this discussion regarding different signalling pathways induced by different platelet activating stimuli we now turn to the functional consequences of this diversity. It is well-known that the combined actions of platelet activators often induce synergistic effects. Several studies claim that this synergy/potentiation demands simultaneous signalling through both G_q and G_i. As described above, ADP activates platelets through the G_q-coupled P2Y1-receptor and the G_i-coupled P2Y12-receptor. The importance of simultaneous G_q and G_i-signalling have been shown in experiments using selective receptor antagonists. Selective blockade of the G_i-coupled P2Y12-receptor inhibited ADP-induced platelet aggregation but was reversed by addition of epinephrine [25]. Likewise, serotonin acting through G_q reversed the inhibiting effect on ADP-induced aggregation exerted by blockade of the G_q-coupled P2Y1-receptor. It was also shown that serotonin and epinephrine were without effect when added alone but induced platelet aggregation when combined. All those experiments clearly show that simultaneous G_q and G_i signalling is essential for effective platelet activation. Synergistic effects of epinephrine combined with the thromboxane mimetic U46619 further confirm the importance of concomitant G_i and G_q-signalling [26]. In cases when U46619 appear to induce platelet aggregation on its own it is actually dependent on G_i-signalling from secreted ADP and epinephrine [4]. It has also been suggested that collagen-induced activation of the intracellular protein ERK2 is dependent on ADP-signalling through the G_i-coupled P2Y12 and G_q-coupled TXA_2-signalling [27]. More detailed experiments have investigated synergism between the G_i-signalling pathway and different parts of G_q-signalling. G_q-signalling results in both increased amount of $[Ca^{2+}]_i$ and activation of PKC.

U46619-induced platelet aggregation was inhibited with a PKC-blocker, but restored by selective G_i-stimulation [28]. Likewise, when inhibiting intracellular Ca^{2+}-rises, supplemental G_i-stimulation was necessary for U46619-induced aggregation. Thus, G_i-activation can synergize with selective parts of G_q-stimulation. The complexity of potentiating effects of different platelet activators can be further acknowledged by recent findings suggesting that the G_q-signalling pathway can be substituted for by other pathways. Experiments performed on G_q-deficient mice show that simultaneous signalling through G_i and $G_{12/13}$ is sufficient to induce platelet aggregation [29]. This cooperation between G_i and $G_{12/13}$ have also been observed on human platelets [30]. Furthermore, synergistic effects occur on human platelets between thrombopoietin and selective G_i-stimulation by ADP in the presence of a P2Y1-inhibitor [31]. Interestingly, the effect induced by thrombopoietin and G_i-stimulation was not dependent on G_q-signalling since there were no intracellular Ca^{2+}-increase. However, the importance of Ca^{2+}-signalling should not be neglected when investigating synergistic effects not involving G_q-stimulation. More studies are needed on this issue since a somewhat paradoxical dependence on intracellular Ca^{2+} was observed in the above mentioned studies [30,31].

Platelet Activation Induced by Epinephrine

Epinephrine is considered to be a weak platelet activator, which especially acts by potentiating the effects of other activators. To name a few, synergistic effects have been observed for epinephrine combined with substances such as thrombin, platelet activating factor (PAF), ADP, lysophosphatidic acid (LPA), estrogens, histamine, serotonin and thrombopoietin [31-38]. Furthermore, we have unpublished observations showing that epinephrine can act in synergy with ristocetin to increase platelet adhesion to surfaces coated with either albumin or collagen (Figure 1). Even though ristocetin is not an endogenous substance it is an interesting experimental molecule since it activates platelets by promoting the interaction between vWf and platelet GPIb-IX-V [39]. This suggests that epinephrine might be important for early events in platelet adhesion since binding of vWf to GPIb-IX-V is an initial interaction after vessel injury. Another molecule that needs further attention is LPA. We have previously shown that a synergistic effect of epinephrine and LPA on platelet adhesion is dependent on the presence of ADP [33]. Thus, a complex interaction between three different activators was needed for this effect to appear. We claim that further research is needed in the area of epinephrine and LPA cross-talk since LPA is present in atherosclerotic plaques and might be important for thrombus development after plaque rupture [40].

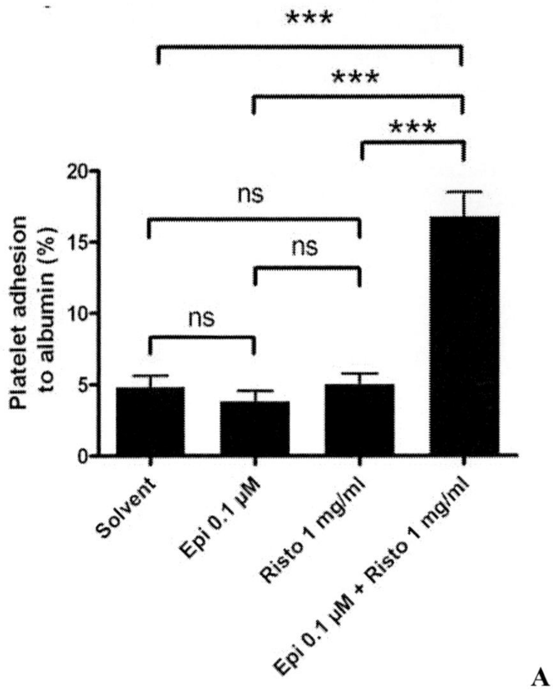

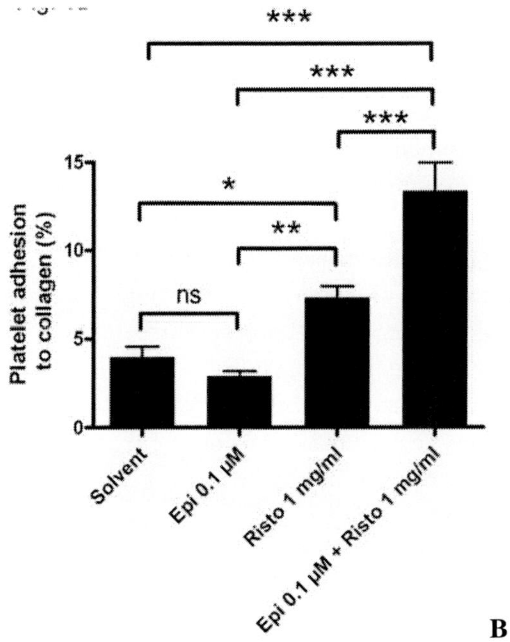

Figure 1. Static adhesion of human platelets to albumin and collagen was measured with a previously described assay [23,33]. Briefly, platelets in plasma from healthy volunteers were incubated with epinephrine (Epi) and/or ristocetin (Risto) in 96-well microplates coated with albumin (Figure 1A) or collagen (Figure 1B). Adhered platelets were detected enzymatically and quantified by spectrophotometry. The figure shows that epinephrine act in synergy with ristocetin to increase platelet adhesion to albumin and collagen (n=30). Experiments were performed in the absence of externally added magnesium. This explains the low basal adhesion to collagen, which is elevated in the presence of magnesium [23]. Results are presented as mean+SEM. *$p<0.05$, **$p<0.01$, ***$p<0.001$, ns = not significant.

The dependence on co-stimulation with one or even two other activators in order to measure effects of epinephrine makes it especially complicated to elucidate which intracellular pathways are activated by epinephrine. In some experiments the results observed are probably not the result of epinephrine stimulation *per se* but instead the combined effect of epinephrine and trace amounts of other substances. Different signalling pathways have been proposed for epinephrine-induced platelet activation (Figure 2). First of all, α_{2A}-adrenergic receptors are G-protein coupled. Activation of G-proteins in general results in dissociation of the G-protein into one α- and one $\beta\gamma$-subunit. Both, the α- and the $\beta\gamma$-subunits are able to stimulate intracellular signalling, which will be discussed below in the context of epinephrine. G-proteins can also be classified into different subtypes. Results from a study on mice has shown that the G-protein coupled to α_{2A}-adrenergic receptors is a specific kind of G_i-protein called G_z [41], which is a known inhibitor of cAMP accumulation [42]. Epinephrine potentiated the platelet aggregating effect of ADP, serotonin, U46619, collagen and the PAR4 (thrombin receptor) peptide agonist GYPGQV in wild-type mice, while the effect was decreased or absent in $G\alpha_z$(-/-) mice [41]. Furthermore, epinephrine was less potent in reducing cAMP-levels after stimulation with PGI_2 in the $G\alpha_z$(-/-) mice. $G\alpha_z$(-/-) mice were also less prone to develop thromboembolism *in vivo* after injection with collagen and epinephrine. Further support for G_z and not other G_i-proteins in epinephrine-induced platelet responses comes from a study on mice lacking $G\alpha_{i2}$, which show normal inhibition of adenylyl cyclase by epinephrine [43]. Although the importance of G_z for epinephrine-induced platelet activation has only been shown in mice it is likely that the same is true for humans since human platelets also contain G_z [44]. As evident from the above discussion, it is generally assumed that G_z inhibits adenylyl cyclase, which results in decreased amounts of cAMP leading to platelet activation. In turn, results from several studies have shown that epinephrine is not able to activate platelets by elevation of $[Ca^{2+}]_i$ [34,45-47]. Also, early studies have reported that epinephrine by itself is unable to induce production of DAG [48] and IP_3 [47] and is consequently not able to activate PLC. Since DAG, IP_3 and PLC are signalling molecules necessary for elevation of $[Ca^{2+}]_i$, these results further confirm the inability of epinephrine to affect Ca^{2+}-signalling pathways. However, it should be mentioned that when using aequorin as Ca^{2+}-sensor an increase in $[Ca^{2+}]_i$ have been observed [49]. This effect was only seen when extracellular Ca^{2+} was present indicating that epinephrine activates Ca^{2+}-influx. Furthermore, a role for influx of extracellular Ca^{2+} after epinephrine-induced platelet activation have been confirmed by another study [50]. Care must however be exercised when interpreting these results since both studies were performed in the absence of ADP-inhibitors, which makes it impossible to reject that the effect observed were a synergistic effect between adrenaline and trace amounts of ADP. Consequently, there is a lot of evidence showing that epinephrine by itself cannot increase $[Ca^{2+}]_i$. However, it can potentiate the Ca^{2+}-elevating capacity of other platelet agonists [45,46]. This effect of epinephrine was proposed to be the result of cAMP-mediated modulation of Ca^{2+}-signalling [45]. However, the role of cAMP in epinephrine signalling has been questioned. Even though it has been found that epinephrine can decrease basal cAMP-levels [45], others have shown that epinephrine only decrease levels of cAMP in platelets where cAMP-levels are pre-elevated by PGI_2 [51]. Furthermore, addition of an adenylyl cyclase inhibitor could not reverse the defective epinephrine signalling in $G\alpha_z$ (-/-) mice. It is therefore possible that other signalling pathways than adenylyl cyclase inhibition contribute to epinephrine induced platelet activation. Another interesting intracellular signalling molecule is the Ras-protein Rap1b, which is involved in activation of the $\alpha_{IIb}\beta_3$-integrin [52]. Activation of Rap1b induced by epinephrine was shown to be dependent on phosphoinositide 3-kinase (PI3K), but independent of cAMP [53]. These results favour the view of cAMP as a modulator with none or only a minor role in epinephrine induced signalling. Instead it suggests a role for PI3K, of which three different isoforms (α, β, γ) are present in platelets [54]. Two of the isoforms, PI3Kγ and PI3Kβ, are known to interact with $\beta\gamma$-subunits from G-proteins, which results in the formation of phosphatidylinositol-3,4,5-trisphosphate [PtdIns(3,4,5)P_3] [55]. In turn, PtdIns(3,4,5)P_3 act together with its dephosphorylation product PtdIns(4,5)P_2 as messenger molecules in different signalling pathways [56]. The addition of PtdIns(3,4,5)P_3 to platelets treated with the PI3K inhibitor wortmannin reversed the inhibiting effect of wortmannin on epinephrine induced Rap1b activation [57]. This indicates that activation of Rap1b is a consequence of PtdIns(3,4,5)P_3-activation induced by PI3K. Another molecule coupled to the PI3K pathway by its ability to be activated by PtdIns(3,4,5)P_3 and PtdIns(3,4)P_2 is Akt [57]. Similarly to Rap1b, Akt-signalling is able to activate platelets by its effect on integrin function [58]. Activation of this molecule through stimulation of the G_i-coupled P2Y12-receptor can be substituted for by epinephrine [59]. This observed activation of Akt was only present when epinephrine was combined with other activators and was not an effect of epinephrine *per se*. Furthermore, it is not impossible that ADP-signalling through G_i-proteins contributed to the epinephrine induced Rap1b activation observed by Woulfe *et al* [53]. This would imply that epinephrine induced activation of Akt and Rap1b is the result of co-stimulation with other activators. Whether this is the case or not must be addressed in future studies. Nevertheless, the ability of epinephrine to affect both Akt and Rap1b, which both are downstream of PI3K suggests an important role for the $\beta\gamma$-subunit of G_z for epinephrine signalling. However, it must also be stressed that there are other possible ways for epinephrine to activate Rap1b, which may or may not be connected to PI3K. An early study have suggested that the effect of epinephrine on Rap1b is mediated through reduction of the activity of Rap1b.GAP, which normally acts to inactivate Rap1b [60]. This would result in prolonged activity of Rap1b. Furthermore, Rap1, Rap1.GAP and $G\alpha_z$ can associate in a ternary complex [61]. This observation is interesting since it creates a possibility for regulation of Rap1b-activity by the α-subunit of G_z. Other signalling pathways suggested for epinephrine induced platelet activation involve ion channels. Platelet stimulation with epinephrine result in increased levels of intracellular Cl^- [62]. Furthermore, platelet activation in general is connected to increased intracellular pH, which is mostly the result of sodium/hydrogen (Na^+/H^+) exchange [63]. Alkalinization induced by PAF as well as thrombin is potentiated by epinephrine [64,65]. It has been suggested that Na^+/H^+ exchange is important for TXA_2-synthesis at the level of arachidonic acid liberation [66]. The alkalinizing effect of epinephrine has further been shown to be dependent on fibrinogen, ADP and the TXA_2-producing cyclooxygenase system [67]. Those studies further acknowledge the importance of co-stimulation for epinephrine-induced effects. Further research is needed to elucidate the specific role of these ion channel events in epinephrine induced platelet activation. More research is also needed concerning the role of TXA_2. Secondary platelet aggregation induced by epinephrine has been observed to be dependent on released TXA_2 [66]. However, whether this is an effect of epinephrine *per se* or not is uncertain.

In conclusion, epinephrine cannot by itself activate platelets by increasing $[Ca^{2+}]_i$. It can decrease the levels of cAMP but the significance of this for platelet activation has been questioned. Probably, epinephrine activates the Gβγ-PI3K-pathway, but further research is needed to conclude whether this is an effect of epinephrine *per se* or not.

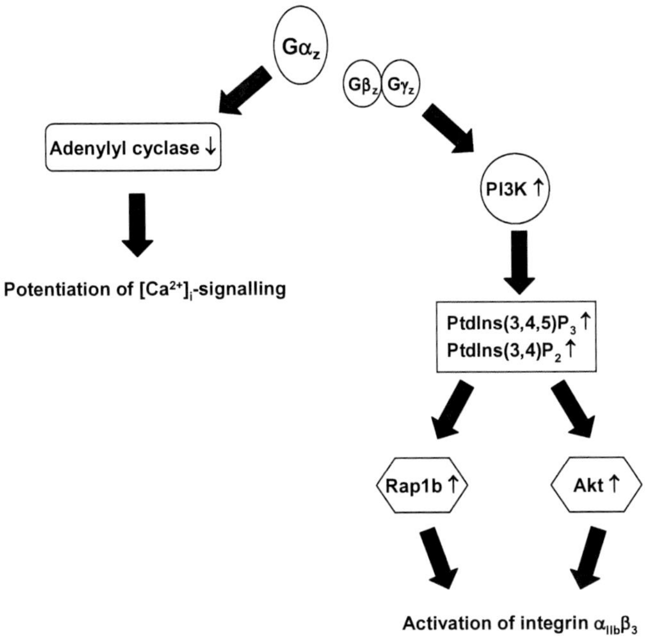

Figure 2. The figure shows a simplified view of intracellular signalling pathways induced by the binding of epinephrine to α_{2A}-ARs. Probably, other less well described pathways further contribute to epinephrine induced platelet activation (see text). Signalling through β_2-ARs is omitted from the figure.

Individual Variability

A high degree of inter-individual variability has been shown for the platelet activating effect of epinephrine. In a study performed on 140 healthy subjects, 16% were classified as non-responders to epinephrine having minimal aggregation without secondary aggregation to 100 μmol/L epinephrine [68]. Furthermore, a smaller study reported 20% of healthy volunteers as non-responders to epinephrine-induced aggregation in platelet rich plasma [69]. The cause of this heterogeneity is not established but different mechanisms have been proposed. Interestingly, the adenylyl cyclase-cAMP system seem to be equally effective in responders and non-responders to epinephrine [70-72] further questioning the role of this pathway in epinephrine-induced platelet activation. Studies investigating the influence of α_{2A}-AR density have shown inconsistent results. Kambayashi *et al* reported decreased levels of α_{2A}-ARs with unchanged binding affinity in non-responders [68]. In contrast, Nakahashi *et al* found no difference in the number of α_{2A}-ARs while the binding affinity was significantly decreased for non-responders [70]. Regarding α_{2A}-AR-genotype, 16 variants have been found and this genetic polymorphism have been shown to be relevant for platelet function [73,74]. Furthermore, one possible explanation for the occurrence of the non-responsive state is lack of PLA_2-activation in the presence of epinephrine combined with fibrinogen [71]. The studies described above by Kambayashi *et al* [68] and Pyo *et al* [69] were both performed in Asian countries and the authors suggested that non-response could be a "racial" trait. However, we have observed huge variations in epinephrine-induced platelet adhesion in Caucasians suggesting that this is a general phenomenon (Figure 3). We speculate that the individual variation observed with epinephrine is just the result of the normal variation that is observed with all biological events. What makes epinephrine special are the observations of total lack of response for non-responders and not just different degrees of efficiency. However, since epinephrine is a weak agonist it is possible that the apparent non-response could be eliminated with the use of more sensitive assays. It is also possible that epinephrine non-response could be overcome if experimental conditions are optimized for factors important for epinephrine-induced platelet activation.

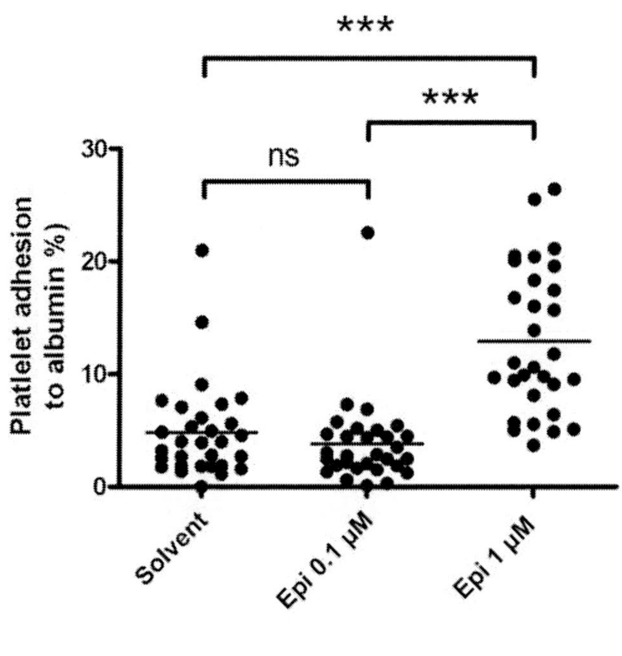

Figure 3. Static adhesion of human platelets to albumin was measured with a previously described assay [23,33]. Briefly, platelets in plasma from healthy volunteers were incubated with epinephrine (Epi) in 96-well microplates coated with albumin. Adhered platelets were detected enzymatically and quantified by spectrophotometry. The figure shows that platelet adhesion to albumin is increased by 1 µM epinephrine (n=30). The increase was highly donor-dependent. ***$p<0.001$, ns = not significant.

Epinephrine, Platelets, Stress and Cardiovascular Disease

Cardiovascular disease (CVD) is the major cause of mortality and morbidity in the western world, with acute myocardial infarction (AMI) accounting for a large part of that observed [75]. The aetiology of AMI is usually a chronic and multi-factorial process, with several risk factors such as elevated serum cholesterol, hypertension and smoking, being well recognised. In addition to established risk factors, numerous studies are today available that points towards psychological stress as an important factor for acute cardiovascular events, such as AMI, left-ventricular dysfunction or dysrhytmia; as well as the chronic atherosclerotic process [76]. The case-control INTERHEART study, showed that people from 52 countries with AMI reported higher prevalence of stress at work or at home, socioeconomic stress, and major life events in the past year [77]. The results suggested that, in both men and women of various ages, psychosocial stress accounted for as much as 30% of the attributable risk of AMI. In fact, since men with lower socioeconomical status were found to have more leukocyte-platelet aggregates in blood, it was suggested that platelet activation is a mechanism through which social position influences cardiovascular risk [78]. In addition, approximately 4% of AMI might be caused by heavy physical activity and the risk are reported to be more than 100 times greater for individuals who are habitually sedentary [79].

Thus, lifestyle and daily situations, such as psychological stress and heavy physical activity, that are associated to actions of epinephrine [80], may act as triggers for acute coronary syndrome (ACS) and some other associations are: 1) intense anger, fear, anxiety are associated with acute manifestation of ACS [81,82]; 2) plasma epinephrine and norepinephrine levels are increased upon AMI [83]; 3) increasing catecholamine concentrations are associated with both ACS and cerebrovascular events during the morning hours [84-90]; and 4) ADP- and epinephrine-induced platelet aggregability increase during active morning hours but not when subjects remain supine and inactive [91-93]. The circadian pattern of both AMI and sudden cardiac death with a peak in the morning hours has also been found in a meta-analysis [94]. In addition to increased catecholamines in the morning, peak corticotropin and cortisol concentrations occur in the early morning [88]. However, in contrast to the large amount of studies that show weak but distinct effects of epinephrine on platelets, only few studies report effects of cortisol on platelets. Furthermore, the effects reported are minor. A recent study showed that administration of hydrocortisone decreased the platelet expression of GPIb (of the GPIb-IX-V complex) whereas the expression of P-selectin, α_{IIb} (of the $\alpha_{IIb}\beta_3$ integrin) and activated $\alpha_{IIb}\beta_3$ receptors was unchanged [95]. In contrast to most other external platelet membrane proteins, expression of GPIb decrease upon activation because this protein is redistributed into intracellular compartments [96].

Also glucagon has been related to stress and intravenous glucagon has been reported to increase ADP-induced platelet aggregation [97]. In a randomized placebo-controlled study by Rosenfeld *et al* 1994, volunteers that received stress hormone infusion (epinephrine, cortisol, or glucagon) for 24 h showed increased circulating fibrinogen concentrations, weakly increased ex vivo collagen-induced platelet aggregation and dense granule release [98]. There was no change in the placebo group. In a more recent blind placebo-controlled cross-over study also by Rosenfeld *et al* 1998, a stress hormone cocktail administered intravenously for 24 h (epinephrine, cortisol, glucagon, angiotensin II and vasopressin) was reported to cause thrombocytosis but not affect platelet aggregation induced by collagen, ADP or ristocetin [99]. Conversely, the stress hormone cocktail caused increased fibrinolytic and anticoagulant activity. Epinephrine is likely capable to cause thrombocytosis since studies using infusion of epinephrine [100] as well as experimentally induced acute physiological stress [101] or exercise [102-104] are reported to increase platelet count. However, the exercise-induced increase of platelet count are dependent on age and sedentary lifestyle [105] and increased platelet count is also often accompanied by increased white as well as red blood cell count [102,103]. In a recent systematic review by Thrall *et al* 2007 [106] it was concluded that acute stress increased the fibrinogen and vWf levels significantly in the majority of the studies. Thrall *et al* did also conclude that the greatest risk of stress-induced thrombogenesis occurs in the period immediately after physical activity or psychological stress, rather than during the activity. In conclusion, studies of acute stress on platelet effects have generally shown increased secretion of platelet specific products as well as increased platelet aggregation [106].

In contrast to acute stress, which appears to trigger acute thrombotic and other cardiovascular events, chronic stress appears to affect cardiovascular risk mainly by accelerating the atherosclerotic process [76]. Indices of chronic emotional and psychosocial stress are depression, chronic anxiety, sleep deprivation and work-related stress. Depressive symptoms are common in coronary artery disease patients and are associated with increased cardiac risk as well as sudden death and all-cause mortality [76,107,108] but the underlying pathophysiological mechanisms are poorly understood. Several possible mechanisms for this association have been reviewed by Shimbo *et al* 2005 [109], and one of them is that platelet α_2-ARs are supersensitive in patients with depression [110,111]. Furthermore, a study by Wenneberg *et al* 1997 suggests that modes of anger expression may be associated with increased collagen-induced platelet aggregation [112]. As reviewed by Brotman *et al* 2007, there are several studies that show correlations with angry and hostile temperament as well as personality type D (distressed) and A (anxiety/hypervigilance) with cardiovascular death and ischaemic heart disease [76]. Regarding work-related stress there are few associations with platelets reported. One recent study report that after adjusting for conventional CVD risk factors, such as age, sex, smoking, hypertension, diabetes, hypercholesterolaemia, obesity, alcohol drinking, regular exercise, and sociodemographics, long driving time for professional drivers was still associated with significant increased platelet count [113].

The mechanisms for increased thrombotic risk and accelerating atherosclerotic process upon chronic stress are most probably several. Upon chronic stress, the fluctations in stress hormones, can damage the hemostatic homeostasis by repeated enhancement of platelet activity during, in many cases, daily stress. This may accelerate the atherosclerotic process and thereby exposing individuals to risks of cardiovascular events. A similar process is also suggested to accelerate vascular injury, organ damage and cardiovascular complications induced by hypertension [114-116] and diabetes [117-120].

An important question to be asked is if the synergistic effects of epinephrine observed in several *in vitro* studies, as discussed earlier in this review, are associated with findings including factors acting *in vivo.* Such factors are for example mental stress, hypertension and smoking. Epinephrine has been shown to potentiate ADP-induced aggregation after experimentally induced mental stress [121]. Furthermore, platelet aggregation induced by ADP or serotonin as well as β-thromboglobulin (β-TG) has been found to increase more in the advanced phase of hypertension than in the early phase of hypertension after mental stress [116]. These studies show that mental stress increases both synergistic platelet mechanisms of activation as well as pathological influences. Such continuous enhancement of platelet activation is very likely to accelerate vascular as well as end-organ damage and cause thrombosis. Another factor, which is clearly established as a major risk for atherothrombosis, is cigarette smoking. Also in this case epinephrine appears important since platelet aggregability induced by epinephrine, as well as ADP, is enhanced in habitual smokers [122].

Cohen and McCombs did already 1967 and 1968 report that experimentally induced thrombocytosis in rabbits was associated with accelerated atherosclerotic process whereas experimental thrombocytopenia prevented atherosclerosis [123,124]. Then, the participation of platelet derived growth factor in the initiation of atherosclerosis was emphasized by Ross et al 1982 [125]. The central mechanism of the pathogenesis of atherosclerosis was later on called "the response to injury" hypothesis by Ross 1993 [126]. Recent studies have established platelets as major players, not only in thrombosis formation, but also in initiation of the atherogenetic process [127,128]. The "response to injury" hypothesis defined that atherosclerosis is a normal response to arterial injury where the injurious triggering effects are abnormally prolonged or amplified, or the capacity to resist the injurious triggers is weakened. One such trigger might be epinephrine in various conditions of stress. In early studies platelets were reported to take up epinephrine from the surroundings and thereafter release it [3,129]. The uptake was proportional to the concentration in plasma. Since the plasma concentration of epinephrine, as been discussed earlier in this paper, increase both upon acute and chronic stress the platelet uptake will most probably increase dose-dependently to stress. Consequently, when platelets take up more epinephrine they are also capable to secrete more epinephrine locally upon activation. As also been discussed earlier in the present paper, epinephrine, derived from platelets as well as from adrenal glands, can synergistically increase the activating properties of almost every other known platelet activator. In fact, signalling initiated by epinephrine through α_2-ARs on the platelet surface has recently been shown to significantly contribute to thrombus stabilization *in vivo* [130]. Increased plasma levels of epinephrine, upon acute as well as chronic stress, may thus cause increased uptake by platelets and increased release upon activation leading to synergistic enhancement of platelet activation and increased risk of thrombosis. Through this quite unique mechanism, epinephrine might be a cornerstone in the pathogenesis of atherosclerosis and thrombosis. The importance of other stress hormones regarding their direct effects on platelets remains to be elucidated further.

Conclusion

Epinephrine is a weak platelet activator that induces its effects through binding to α_{2A}-ARs. The weak effect makes epinephrine important as a potentiator of other platelet activating events. This is evident from *in vitro* studies where several different platelet activators have been shown to act synergistic when combined with epinephrine. Detailed knowledge about the intracellular signalling pathways induced by epinephrine is scarce and need further investigation. Especially interesting is the PI3K-pathway induced by the βγ-subunit of G-proteins. In a pathophysiological context there is a clear connection between epinephrine and conditions like stress and atherosclerosis. However, the extent to which this association can explain cardiovascular events must be further investigated.

Acknowledgements

This work was financed by the Cardiovascular Inflammation Research Centre at Linköping University, Sweden.

References

[1] Gibbins JM. Platelet adhesion signalling and the regulation of thrombus formation. *J Cell Sci* 2004; 117:3415-3425.

[2] Ruggeri ZM. Platelets in atherothrombosis. *Nat Med* 2002; 8:1227-1234.

[3] Born GV, Smith JB. Uptake, metabolism and release of (3H)-adrenaline by human platelets. *Br J Pharmacol* 1970; 39:765-778.

[4] Paul BZ, Jin J, Kunapuli SP. Molecular mechanism of thromboxane A(2)-induced platelet aggregation. Essential role for p2t(ac) and alpha(2a) receptors. *J Biol Chem* 1999; 274:29108-29114.

[5] O'Brien JR. Some Effects of Adrenaline and Anti-Adrenaline Compounds on Platelets in Vitro and in Vivo. *Nature* 1963; 200:763-764.

[6] Hsu CY, Knapp DR, Halushka PV. The effects of alpha adrenergic agents on human platelet aggregation. *J Pharmacol Exp Ther* 1979; 208:366-370.

[7] Grant JA, Scrutton MC. Interaction of selective alpha-adrenoceptor agonists and antagonists with human and rabbit blood platelets. *Br J Pharmacol* 1980; 71:121-134.

[8] Hoffman BB, De Lean A, Wood CL, Schocken DD, Lefkowitz RJ. Alpha-adrenergic receptor subtypes: quantitative assessment by ligand binding. *Life Sci* 1979; 24:1739-1745.

[9] Kobilka BK, Matsui H, Kobilka TS, Yang-Feng TL, Francke U, Caron MG, et al. Cloning, sequencing, and expression of the gene coding for the human platelet alpha 2-adrenergic receptor. *Science* 1987; 238:650-656.

[10] Civantos Calzada B, Aleixandre de Artinano A. Alpha-adrenoceptor subtypes. *Pharmacol Res* 2001; 44:195-208.

[11] Mills DC, Smith JB. The influence on platelet aggregation of drugs that affect the accumulation of adenosine 3':5'-cyclic monophosphate in platelets. *Biochem J* 1971; 121:185-196.

[12] Jakobs KH, Saur W, Schultz G. Characterization of alpha- and beta-adrenergic receptors linked to human platelet adenylate cyclase. *Naunyn Schmiedebergs Arch Pharmacol* 1978; 302:285-291.

[13] Kerry R, Scrutton MC. Platelet beta-adrenoceptors. *Br J Pharmacol* 1983; 79:681-691.

[14] Haslam RJ, Taylor A. Effects of catecholamines on the formation of adenosine 3':5'-cyclic monophosphate in human blood platelets. *Biochem J* 1971; 125:377-379.

[15] Kerry R, Scrutton MC, Wallis RB. Mammalian platelet adrenoceptors. *Br J Pharmacol* 1984; 81:91-102.

[16] Larsson PT, Wallen NH, Martinsson A, Egberg N, Hjemdahl P. Significance of platelet beta-adrenoceptors for platelet responses in vivo and in vitro. *Thromb Haemost* 1992; 68:687-693.

[17] Anfossi G, Russo I, Massucco P, Mattiello L, Trovati M. Catecholamines, via beta-adrenoceptors, increase intracellular concentrations of 3',5'-cyclic guanosine monophosphate (cGMP) through nitric oxide in human platelets. *Thromb Haemost* 2002; 87:539-540.

[18] Hjemdahl P, Larsson PT, Wallen NH. Effects of stress and beta-blockade on platelet function. *Circulation* 1991; 84:VI44-61.

[19] Lechin F, van der Dijs B, Lechin A, Orozco B, Lechin M, Baez S, et al. Plasma neurotransmitters and cortisol in chronic illness: role of stress. *J Med* 1994; 25:181-192.

[20] Wang JS, Cheng LJ. Effect of strenuous, acute exercise on alpha2-adrenergic agonist-potentiated platelet activation. *Arterioscler Thromb Vasc Biol* 1999; 19:1559-1565.

[21] Dimsdale JE, Moss J. Plasma catecholamines in stress and exercise. *JAMA* 1980; 243:340-342.

[22] Graff J, Klinkhardt U, Harder S. Pharmacodynamic profile of antiplatelet agents: marked differences between single versus costimulation with platelet activators. *Thromb Res* 2004; 113:295-302.

[23] Eriksson AC, Whiss PA. Measurement of adhesion of human platelets in plasma to protein surfaces in microplates. *J Pharmacol Toxicol Methods* 2005; 52:356-365.

[24] Woulfe DS. Platelet G protein-coupled receptors in hemostasis and thrombosis. *J Thromb Haemost* 2005; 3:2193-2200.

[25] Jin J, Kunapuli SP. Coactivation of two different G protein-coupled receptors is essential for ADP-induced platelet aggregation. *Proc Natl Acad Sci U S A* 1998; 95:8070-8074.

[26] Pulcinelli FM, Pesciotti M, Pignatelli P, Riondino S, Gazzaniga PP. Concomitant activation of Gi and Gq protein-coupled receptors does not require an increase in cytosolic calcium for platelet aggregation. *FEBS Lett* 1998; 435:115-118.

[27] Roger S, Pawlowski M, Habib A, Jandrot-Perrus M, Rosa JP, Bryckaert M. Costimulation of the Gi-coupled ADP receptor and the Gq-coupled TXA2 receptor is required for ERK2 activation in collagen-induced platelet aggregation. *FEBS Lett* 2004; 556:227-235.

[28] Quinton TM, Kim S, Dangelmaier C, Dorsam RT, Jin J, Daniel JL, et al. Protein kinase C- and calcium-regulated pathways independently synergize with Gi pathways in agonist-induced fibrinogen receptor activation. *Biochem J* 2002; 368:535-543.

[29] Nieswandt B, Schulte V, Zywietz A, Gratacap MP, Offermanns S. Costimulation of Gi- and G12/G13-mediated signaling pathways induces integrin alphaIIbbeta3 activation in platelets. *J Biol Chem* 2002; 277:39493-39498.
[30] Dorsam RT, Kim S, Jin J, Kunapuli SP. Coordinated signaling through both G12/13 and G(i) pathways is sufficient to activate GPIIb/IIIa in human platelets. *J Biol Chem* 2002; 277:47588-47595.
[31] Campus F, Lova P, Bertoni A, Sinigaglia F, Balduini C, Torti M. Thrombopoietin complements G(i)- but not G(q)-dependent pathways for integrin alphaIIbbeta3 activation and platelet aggregation. *J Biol Chem* 2005; 280:24386-24395.
[32] Steen VM, Holmsen H, Aarbakke G. The platelet-stimulating effect of adrenaline through alpha 2-adrenergic receptors requires simultaneous activation by a true stimulatory platelet agonist. Evidence that adrenaline per se does not induce human platelet activation in vitro. *Thromb Haemost* 1993; 70:506-513.
[33] Eriksson AC, Whiss PA, Nilsson UK. Adhesion of human platelets to albumin is synergistically increased by lysophosphatidic acid and adrenaline in a donor-dependent fashion. *Blood Coagul Fibrinolysis* 2006; 17:359-368.
[34] Nilsson UK, Svensson SP, Grenegard M. Synergistic activation of human platelets by lysophosphatidic acid and adrenaline. *Haematologica* 2002; 87:730-739; discussion 739.
[35] Haseruck N, Erl W, Pandey D, Tigyi G, Ohlmann P, Ravanat C, et al. The plaque lipid lysophosphatidic acid stimulates platelet activation and platelet-monocyte aggregate formation in whole blood: involvement of P2Y1 and P2Y12 receptors. *Blood* 2004; 103:2585-2592.
[36] Akarasereenont P, Tripatara P, Chotewuttakorn S, Palo T, Thaworn A. The effects of estrone, estradiol and estriol on platelet aggregation induced by adrenaline and adenosine diphosphate. *Platelets* 2006; 17:441-447.
[37] Masini E, Di Bello MG, Raspanti S, Fomusi Ndisang J, Baronti R, Cappugi P, et al. The role of histamine in platelet aggregation by physiological and immunological stimuli. *Inflamm Res* 1998; 47:211-220.
[38] Roevens P, De Clerck F, de Chaffoy de Courcelles D. The synergistic effect of 5-hydroxytryptamine and epinephrine on the human platelet is related to the activation of phospholipase C. *Eur J Pharmacol* 1993; 245:273-280.
[39] Coller BS, Peerschke EI, Scudder LE, Sullivan CA. Studies with a murine monoclonal antibody that abolishes ristocetin-induced binding of von Willebrand factor to platelets: additional evidence in support of GPIb as a platelet receptor for von Willebrand factor. *Blood* 1983; 61:99-110.
[40] Siess W. Athero- and thrombogenic actions of lysophosphatidic acid and sphingosine-1-phosphate. *Biochim Biophys Acta* 2002; 1582:204-215.
[41] Yang J, Wu J, Kowalska MA, Dalvi A, Prevost N, O'Brien PJ, et al. Loss of signaling through the G protein, Gz, results in abnormal platelet activation and altered responses to psychoactive drugs. *Proc Natl Acad Sci U S A* 2000; 97:9984-9989.
[42] Wong YH, Conklin BR, Bourne HR. Gz-mediated hormonal inhibition of cyclic AMP accumulation. *Science* 1992; 255:339-342.

[43] Jantzen HM, Milstone DS, Gousset L, Conley PB, Mortensen RM. Impaired activation of murine platelets lacking G alpha(i2). *J Clin Invest* 2001; 108:477-483.
[44] Gagnon AW, Manning DR, Catani L, Gewirtz A, Poncz M, Brass LF. Identification of Gz alpha as a pertussis toxin-insensitive G protein in human platelets and megakaryocytes. *Blood* 1991; 78:1247-1253.
[45] Keularts IM, van Gorp RM, Feijge MA, Vuist WM, Heemskerk JW. alpha(2A)-adrenergic receptor stimulation potentiates calcium release in platelets by modulating cAMP levels. *J Biol Chem* 2000; 275:1763-1772.
[46] Ghilotti M, Lova P, Balduini C, Torti M. Epinephrine induces intracellular Ca2+ mobilization in thrombin-desensitized platelets: a role for GPIb-IX-V. *Platelets* 2007; 18:135-142.
[47] Crouch MF, Lapetina EG. A role for Gi in control of thrombin receptor-phospholipase C coupling in human platelets. *J Biol Chem* 1988; 263:3363-3371.
[48] Siess W, Weber PC, Lapetina EG. Activation of phospholipase C is dissociated from arachidonate metabolism during platelet shape change induced by thrombin or platelet-activating factor. Epinephrine does not induce phospholipase C activation or platelet shape change. *J Biol Chem* 1984; 259:8286-8292.
[49] Ware JA, Johnson PC, Smith M, Salzman EW. Effect of common agonists on cytoplasmic ionized calcium concentration in platelets. Measurement with 2-methyl-6-methoxy 8-nitroquinoline (quin2) and aequorin. *J Clin Invest* 1986; 77:878-886.
[50] Owen NE, Feinberg H, Le Breton GC. Epinephrine induces Ca2+ uptake in human blood platelets. *Am J Physiol* 1980; 239:H483-H488.
[51] Yang J, Wu J, Jiang H, Mortensen R, Austin S, Manning DR, et al. Signaling through Gi family members in platelets. Redundancy and specificity in the regulation of adenylyl cyclase and other effectors. *J Biol Chem* 2002; 277:46035-46042.
[52] Bernardi B, Guidetti GF, Campus F, Crittenden JR, Graybiel AM, Balduini C, et al. The small GTPase Rap1b regulates the cross talk between platelet integrin alpha2beta1 and integrin alphaIIbbeta3. *Blood* 2006; 107:2728-2735.
[53] Woulfe D, Jiang H, Mortensen R, Yang J, Brass LF. Activation of Rap1B by G(i) family members in platelets. *J Biol Chem* 2002; 277:23382-23390.
[54] Hirsch E, Bosco O, Tropel P, Laffargue M, Calvez R, Altruda F, et al. Resistance to thromboembolism in PI3Kgamma-deficient mice. *FASEB J* 2001; 15:2019-2021.
[55] Maier U, Babich A, Nurnberg B. Roles of non-catalytic subunits in gbetagamma-induced activation of class I phosphoinositide 3-kinase isoforms beta and gamma. *J Biol Chem* 1999; 274:29311-29317.
[56] Hawkins PT, Stephens LR. PI3Kgamma is a key regulator of inflammatory responses and cardiovascular homeostasis. *Science* 2007; 318:64-66.
[57] Lova P, Paganini S, Hirsch E, Barberis L, Wymann M, Sinigaglia F, et al. A selective role for phosphatidylinositol 3,4,5-trisphosphate in the Gi-dependent activation of platelet Rap1B. *J Biol Chem* 2003; 278:131-138.
[58] Yin H, Stojanovic A, Hay N, Du X. The role of Akt in the signaling pathway of the glycoprotein Ib-IX-induced platelet activation. *Blood* 2007;
[59] Kim S, Jin J, Kunapuli SP. Akt activation in platelets depends on Gi signaling pathways. *J Biol Chem* 2004; 279:4186-4195.

[60] Marti KB, Lapetina EG. Epinephrine suppresses rap1B.GAP-activated GTPase activity in human platelets. *Proc Natl Acad Sci U S A* 1992; 89:2784-2788.

[61] Meng J, Glick JL, Polakis P, Casey PJ. Functional interaction between Galpha(z) and Rap1GAP suggests a novel form of cellular cross-talk. *J Biol Chem* 1999; 274:36663-36669.

[62] Spalding A, Vaitkevicius H, Dill S, MacKenzie S, Schmaier A, Lockette W. Mechanism of epinephrine-induced platelet aggregation. *Hypertension* 1998; 31:603-607.

[63] Rosskopf D. Sodium-hydrogen exchange and platelet function. *J Thromb Thrombolysis* 1999; 8:15-24.

[64] Nieuwland R, Siffert W, Akkerman JW. Effect of epinephrine on the regulation of Na+/H+ exchange in human platelets. *Biochim Biophys Acta* 1993; 1148:185-190.

[65] Steen VM, Cook CA, Tysnes OB, Holmsen H. Potentiation by adrenaline of thrombin-induced elevation of pHi is not essential for synergistic activation of human platelets. *FEBS Lett* 1989; 250:211-214.

[66] Sweatt JD, Johnson SL, Cragoe EJ, Limbird LE. Inhibitors of Na+/H+ exchange block stimulus-provoked arachidonic acid release in human platelets. Selective effects on platelet activation by epinephrine, ADP, and lower concentrations of thrombin. *J Biol Chem* 1985; 260:12910-12919.

[67] Banga HS, Simons ER, Brass LF, Rittenhouse SE. Activation of phospholipases A and C in human platelets exposed to epinephrine: role of glycoproteins IIb/IIIa and dual role of epinephrine. *Proc Natl Acad Sci U S A* 1986; 83:9197-9201.

[68] Kambayashi J, Shinoki N, Nakamura T, Ariyoshi H, Kawasaki T, Sakon M, et al. Prevalence of impaired responsiveness to epinephrine in platelets among Japanese. *Thromb Res* 1996; 81:85-90.

[69] Pyo MK, Yun-Choi HS, Hong YJ. Apparent heterogeneous responsiveness of human platelet rich plasma to catecholamines. *Platelets* 2003; 14:171-178.

[70] Nakahashi TK, Kambayashi J, Nakamura T, Le SN, Yoshitake M, Tandon NN, et al. Platelets in nonresponders to epinephrine stimulation showed reduced response to ADP. *Thromb Res* 2001; 104:127-135.

[71] Nakamura T, Ariyoshi H, Kambayashi J, Ikeda M, Shinoki N, Kawasaki T, et al. Signal transduction system in epinephrine stimulated platelets; comparison between epinephrine sensitive and insensitive platelets. *Thromb Res* 1997; 85:83-93.

[72] Rao AK, Willis J, Kowalska MA, Wachtfogel YT, Colman RW. Differential requirements for platelet aggregation and inhibition of adenylate cyclase by epinephrine. Studies of a familial platelet alpha 2-adrenergic receptor defect. *Blood* 1988; 71:494-501.

[73] Yabe M, Matsubara Y, Takahashi S, Ishihara H, Shibano T, Miyaki K, et al. Identification of ADRA2A polymorphisms related to shear-mediated platelet function. *Biochem Biophys Res Commun* 2006; 347:1001-1005.

[74] Freeman K, Farrow S, Schmaier A, Freedman R, Schork T, Lockette W. Genetic polymorphism of the alpha 2-adrenergic receptor is associated with increased platelet aggregation, baroreceptor sensitivity, and salt excretion in normotensive humans. *Am J Hypertens* 1995; 8:863-869.

[75] Michaud CM, Murray CJ, Bloom BR. Burden of disease--implications for future research. *JAMA* 2001; 285:535-539.
[76] Brotman DJ, Golden SH, Wittstein IS. The cardiovascular toll of stress. *Lancet* 2007; 370:1089-1100.
[77] Rosengren A, Hawken S, Ounpuu S, Sliwa K, Zubaid M, Almahmeed WA, et al. Association of psychosocial risk factors with risk of acute myocardial infarction in 11119 cases and 13648 controls from 52 countries (the INTERHEART study): case-control study. *Lancet* 2004; 364:953-962.
[78] Steptoe A, Magid K, Edwards S, Brydon L, Hong Y, Erusalimsky J. The influence of psychological stress and socioeconomic status on platelet activation in men. *Atherosclerosis* 2003; 168:57-63.
[79] Mittleman MA, Maclure M, Tofler GH, Sherwood JB, Goldberg RJ, Muller JE. Triggering of acute myocardial infarction by heavy physical exertion. Protection against triggering by regular exertion. Determinants of Myocardial Infarction Onset Study Investigators. *N Engl J Med* 1993; 329:1677-1683.
[80] Wortsman J. Role of epinephrine in acute stress. *Endocrinol Metab Clin North Am* 2002; 31:79-106.
[81] Mittleman MA, Maclure M, Sherwood JB, Mulry RP, Tofler GH, Jacobs SC, et al. Triggering of acute myocardial infarction onset by episodes of anger. Determinants of Myocardial Infarction Onset Study Investigators. *Circulation* 1995; 92:1720-1725.
[82] Verrier RL, Mittelman MA. Cardiovascular consequences of anger and other stress states. *Baillieres Clin Neurol* 1997; 6:245-259.
[83] Lubbecke F, Zschatzsch S, Mitrovic V, Husseini H, Schlepper M, Lasch HG, et al. Catecholamines and thrombocyte alpha 2-adrenoceptors in patients with acute myocardial infarction. *Eur Heart J* 1991; 12:88-91.
[84] Willich SN, Linderer T, Wegscheider K, Leizorovicz A, Alamercery I, Schroder R. Increased morning incidence of myocardial infarction in the ISAM Study: absence with prior beta-adrenergic blockade. ISAM Study Group. *Circulation* 1989; 80:853-858.
[85] Willich SN, Goldberg RJ, Maclure M, Perriello L, Muller JE. Increased onset of sudden cardiac death in the first three hours after awakening. *Am J Cardiol* 1992; 70:65-68.
[86] Panza JA, Epstein SE, Quyyumi AA. Circadian variation in vascular tone and its relation to alpha-sympathetic vasoconstrictor activity. *N Engl J Med* 1991; 325:986-990.
[87] Muller JE. Circadian variation in cardiovascular events. *Am J Hypertens* 1999; 12:35S-42S.
[88] Hojlund K, Wildner-Christensen M, Eshoj O, Skjaerbaek C, Holst JJ, Koldkjaer O, et al. Reference intervals for glucose, beta-cell polypeptides, and counterregulatory factors during prolonged fasting. *Am J Physiol Endocrinol Metab* 2001; 280:E50-58.
[89] Marfella R, Esposito K, Gualdiero P, Guigliano D. Morning blood pressure surge and the risk of stroke. *Circulation* 2003; 108:e110-111; author reply e110-111.

[90] Metoki H, Ohkubo T, Kikuya M, Asayama K, Obara T, Hashimoto J, et al. Prognostic significance for stroke of a morning pressor surge and a nocturnal blood pressure decline: the Ohasama study. *Hypertension* 2006; 47:149-154.
[91] Tofler GH, Brezinski D, Schafer AI, Czeisler CA, Rutherford JD, Willich SN, et al. Concurrent morning increase in platelet aggregability and the risk of myocardial infarction and sudden cardiac death. *N Engl J Med* 1987; 316:1514-1518.
[92] Brezinski DA, Tofler GH, Muller JE, Pohjola-Sintonen S, Willich SN, Schafer AI, et al. Morning increase in platelet aggregability. Association with assumption of the upright posture. *Circulation* 1988; 78:35-40.
[93] Willich SN, Pohjola-Sintonen S, Bhatia SJ, Shook TL, Tofler GH, Muller JE, et al. Suppression of silent ischemia by metoprolol without alteration of morning increase of platelet aggregability in patients with stable coronary artery disease. *Circulation* 1989; 79:557-565.
[94] Cohen MC, Rohtla KM, Lavery CE, Muller JE, Mittleman MA. Meta-analysis of the morning excess of acute myocardial infarction and sudden cardiac death. *Am J Cardiol* 1997; 79:1512-1516.
[95] Schuerholz T, Keil O, Wagner T, Klinzing S, Sumpelmann R, Oberle V, et al. Hydrocortisone does not affect major platelet receptors in inflammation in vitro. *Steroids* 2007; 72:609-613.
[96] Schmitz G, Rothe G, Ruf A, Barlage S, Tschope D, Clemetson KJ, et al. European Working Group on Clinical Cell Analysis: Consensus protocol for the flow cytometric characterisation of platelet function. *Thromb Haemost* 1998; 79:885-896.
[97] Proctor SJ, Davies TF, Oxley A, Jones P, Heath A. Increased platelet aggregation induced by glucagon administration. *Acta Haematol* 1980; 64:6-11.
[98] Rosenfeld BA, Faraday N, Campbell D, Dise K, Bell W, Goldschmidt P. Hemostatic effects of stress hormone infusion. *Anesthesiology* 1994; 81:1116-1126.
[99] Rosenfeld BA, Nguyen ND, Sung I, Faraday N. Neuroendocrine stress hormones do not recreate the postoperative hypercoagulable state. *Anesth Analg* 1998; 86:640-645.
[100] Castro-Faria-Neto HC, Bozza PT, Martins MA, Dias PM, Silva PM, Cordeiro RS. Platelet mobilization induced by PAF and its role in the thrombocytosis triggered by adrenaline in rats. *Thromb Haemost* 1989; 62:1107-1111.
[101] Mundal HH, Rostrup M. Blood platelet responses to laboratory stress in young men. The effect of awareness of high blood pressure. *Am J Hypertens* 1996; 9:12-17.
[102] Gimenez M, Mohan-Kumar T, Humbert JC, De Talance N, Buisine J. Leukocyte, lymphocyte and platelet response to dynamic exercise. Duration or intensity effect? *Eur J Appl Physiol Occup Physiol* 1986; 55:465-470.
[103] Chen HI, Tang YR, Wu HJ, Jen CJ. Effects of acute exercise on bleeding time, bleeding amount and blood cell counts: a comparative study. *Thromb Res* 1989; 55:503-510.
[104] Ersoz G, Zergeroglu AM, Ficicilar H, Ozcan H, Oztekin P, Aytac S, et al. Effect of submaximal and incremental upper extremity exercise on platelet function and the role of blood shear stress. *Thromb Res* 2002; 108:297-301.

[105] Gonzales F, Manas M, Seiquer I, Quiles J, Mataix FJ, Huertas JR, et al. Blood platelet function in healthy individuals of different ages. Effects of exercise and exercise conditioning. *J Sports Med Phys Fitness* 1996; 36:112-116.

[106] Thrall G, Lane D, Carroll D, Lip GY. A systematic review of the effects of acute psychological stress and physical activity on haemorheology, coagulation, fibrinolysis and platelet reactivity: Implications for the pathogenesis of acute coronary syndromes. *Thromb Res* 2007; 120:819-847.

[107] Rozanski A, Blumenthal JA, Kaplan J. Impact of psychological factors on the pathogenesis of cardiovascular disease and implications for therapy. *Circulation* 1999; 99:2192-2217.

[108] Lesperance F, Frasure-Smith N, Juneau M, Theroux P. Depression and 1-year prognosis in unstable angina. *Arch Intern Med* 2000; 160:1354-1360.

[109] Shimbo D, Davidson KW, Haas DC, Fuster V, Badimon JJ. Negative impact of depression on outcomes in patients with coronary artery disease: mechanisms, treatment considerations, and future directions. *J Thromb Haemost* 2005; 3:897-908.

[110] Wolfe N, Cohen BM, Gelenberg AJ. Alpha 2-adrenergic receptors in platelet membranes of depressed patients: increased affinity for 3H-yohimbine. *Psychiatry Res* 1987; 20:107-116.

[111] Mori H, Koyama T, Yamashita I. Platelet alpha-2 adrenergic receptor-mediated phosphoinositide responses in endogenous depression. *Life Sci* 1991; 48:741-748.

[112] Wenneberg SR, Schneider RH, Walton KG, MacLean CR, Levitsky DK, Mandarino JV, et al. Anger expression correlates with platelet aggregation. *Behav Med* 1997; 22:174-177.

[113] Chen JC, Chen YJ, Chang WP, Christiani DC. Long driving time is associated with haematological markers of increased cardiovascular risk in taxi drivers. *Occup Environ Med* 2005; 62:890-894.

[114] Haft JI, Fani K. Stress and the induction of intravascular platelet aggregation in the heart. *Circulation* 1973; 48:164-169.

[115] Julius S. Corcoran Lecture. Sympathetic hyperactivity and coronary risk in hypertension. *Hypertension* 1993; 21:886-893.

[116] Tomoda F, Takata M, Kagitani S, Kinuno H, Yasumoto K, Tomita S, et al. Different platelet aggregability during mental stress in two stages of essential hypertension. *Am J Hypertens* 1999; 12:1063-1070.

[117] Winocour PD. Platelets, vascular disease, and diabetes mellitus. *Can J Physiol Pharmacol* 1994; 72:295-303.

[118] Beckman JA, Creager MA, Libby P. Diabetes and atherosclerosis: epidemiology, pathophysiology, and management. *JAMA* 2002; 287:2570-2581.

[119] Ferroni P, Basili S, Falco A, Davi G. Platelet activation in type 2 diabetes mellitus. *J Thromb Haemost* 2004; 2:1282-1291.

[120] Hansen HR, Wolfs JL, Bruggemann L, Sommeijer DW, Bevers E, Hauer AD, et al. Hyperglycemia accelerates arterial thrombus formation and attenuates the antithrombotic response to endotoxin in mice. *Blood Coagul Fibrinolysis* 2007; 18:627-636.

[121] Larsson PT, Hjemdahl P, Olsson G, Angelin B, Hornstra G. Platelet aggregability in humans: contrasting in vivo and in vitro findings during sympatho-adrenal activation and relationship to serum lipids. *Eur J Clin Invest* 1990; 20:398-405.

[122] Fusegawa Y, Handa S. Platelet aggregation induced by ADP or epinephrine is enhanced in habitual smokers. *Thromb Res* 2000; 97:287-295.

[123] Cohen P, McCombs HL. Platelets and atherogenesis. I. Augmentation of cholesterol atherogenesis in the rabbit by a phlebotomy programme designed to induce thrombocytosis. *Br J Exp Pathol* 1967; 48:346-356.

[124] Cohen P, McCombs HL. Platelets and atherogenesis. 2. Amelioration of cholesterol atherogenesis in rabbits with reduced platelet counts as the result of 32P administration. *J Atheroscler Res* 1968; 8:389-398.

[125] Ross R, Raines E, Bowen-Pope D. Growth factors from platelets, monocytes, and endothelium: their role in cell proliferation. *Ann N Y Acad Sci* 1982; 397:18-24.

[126] Ross R. The pathogenesis of atherosclerosis: a perspective for the 1990s. *Nature* 1993; 362:801-809.

[127] Massberg S, Brand K, Gruner S, Page S, Muller E, Muller I, et al. A critical role of platelet adhesion in the initiation of atherosclerotic lesion formation. *J Exp Med* 2002; 196:887-896.

[128] Huo Y, Schober A, Forlow SB, Smith DF, Hyman MC, Jung S, et al. Circulating activated platelets exacerbate atherosclerosis in mice deficient in apolipoprotein E. *Nat Med* 2003; 9:61-67.

[129] Barthel W, Markwardt F. Aggregation of blood platelets by adrenaline and its uptake. *Biochem Pharmacol* 1975; 24:1903-1904.

[130] Pozgajova M, Sachs UJ, Hein L, Nieswandt B. Reduced thrombus stability in mice lacking the alpha2A-adrenergic receptor. *Blood* 2006; 108:510-514.

In: Research Progress on Epinephrine ISBN: 978-1-60456-443-3
Editors: A. G. Lawson and R. I. Gorman, pp. 95-114

Chapter V

Does Epinephrine Cause Hypertension? – "Epinephrine Hypothesis"

Kazuko Masuo*[*], *Gavin W. Lambert, and Murray D. Esler
Human Neurotransmitter Laboratory, Baker Heart Research Institute,
Melbourne, Australia

Abstract

Epinephrine is a prime mover in the "fight or flight" response. Epinephrine elevates heart rate, reduces blood flow to the skin, increases the production of sweat, and increases vigilances. Epinephrine widens the smaller bronchioles in the lungs, dilates the pupils of the eyes and its action on the liver raises blood-sugar levels by stimulating glucose production. In adipose tissue epinephrine raises blood fatty-acid levels. These effects on the cardiovascular system could perhaps play an important role in the onset and maintenance of hypertension.

Epinephrine accounts for 80%, while norepinephrine accounts for 20% of the total hormone secreted from the adrenal medulla. Several studies have reported that epinephrine can augment neurogenic vasoconstriction, while other investigators have shown that urinary or plasma epinephrine levels are correlated with blood pressure. There is not general agreement on this latter point. In several epidemiological studies of either cross-sectional or a longitudinal design, our findings have demonstrated no relationships between plasma epinephrine levels and blood pressure or heart rate.

The "epinephrine hypothesis" proposes that circulating epinephrine is taken up by sympathetic nerves, thereby promoting norepinephrine release during sympathetic nervous system stimulation. It is suggested that binding of co-released epinephrine to pre-synaptic β-adrenoceptors augments exocytotic release of norepinephrine and contribute to high blood pressure (hypertension). Thus, the "epinephrine hypothesis" might explain how adreno-medullary hormonal system activity can contribute to the

[*] Correspondence: Kazuko Masuo, MD, PhD; Human Neurotransmitter Laboratory, Baker Heart Research Institute, 75 Commercial Road, Melbourne 3004, Australia. Phone: +61-3-8532-1111; Fax: +61-3-8532-1100; E-mail: kmasuo@baker.edu.au

development of essential hypertension by augmenting sympathoneuroral norepinephrine release.

There is evidence that the sympathetic nerves of hypertensive patients release epinephrine as a co-transmitter. In this review, results will be presented which suggest that epinephrine is synthesized *in situ* in sympathetic nerve endings via the action of phenylethanolamine-N-methyltransferase (PNMT), which is induced by chronic mental stress exposure. Accordingly, this represents a biomarker of chronic mental stress, rather than a specific mechanism of hypertension, as suggested by the "epinephrine hypothesis".

Introduction

Epinephrine is important to the body's metabolism, was first extracted from the adrenal glands of animals by Jokichi Takamini in 1901. It was synthesized soon after by Friedrich Stolz (1904). Epinephrine together with norepinephrine is secreted principally by the medulla of the adrenal gland. Elevated secretion of epinephrine elicited by fear or anger results in increased heart rate, reduced blood flow to the skin (vasoconstriction) and to the kidneys (renal arteries), increased cardiac output, and elevated renin release, and increased sodium re-absorption in the kidneys. These reactions are often called the "fight or flight" response, and work in concern to prepare the body for strenuous activity. The effects on the cardiovascular system could perhaps play an important role in the onset and maintenance of hypertension. Further, epinephrine's action on the liver raises blood-sugar levels by stimulating glucose production and its action on adipose tissue raises blood fatty acid levels. These effects on glucose and free fatty acids metabolisms might also be related to the cardiovascular risk associated with obesity. Epinephrine is used medicinally as a stimulant in cardiac arrest, as a vasoconstrictor in shock, as a bronchodilator and antispasmodic in bronchial asthma, and to lower intra-ocular pressure in the treatment of glaucoma. These therapeutic implications might be associated with direct epinephrine effects. Epinephrine might also have indirect cardiovascular effect through its stimulation of norepinephrine released by sympathetic nerves.

Epinephrine facilities noradrenergic transmission by stimulating pre-junctional β-2 adrenoceptors in isolated tissue, healthy animals and humans.[1-6] Given that the affinity of epinephrine for the β2-adrenoceptor is more than 200-fold greater than that of norepinephrine, [7-9] this represents a possibly important physiological role with epinephrine modulating norepinephrine release.

A number of clinical and epidemiological observations show that hypertension is associated with heightened sympathetic nervous system activity (high plasma norepinephrine, high muscle sympathetic nerve activity, high whole-body norepinephrine spillover) [10-22]. However, only a limited number of investigations, some in animal models [23, 24] and others in humans [25-27] have documented an association between plasma epinephrine and hypertension. Other investigators have shown no relationships between epinephrine and blood pressure levels. [28-30] The relationships between epinephrine and hypertension have been discordant.

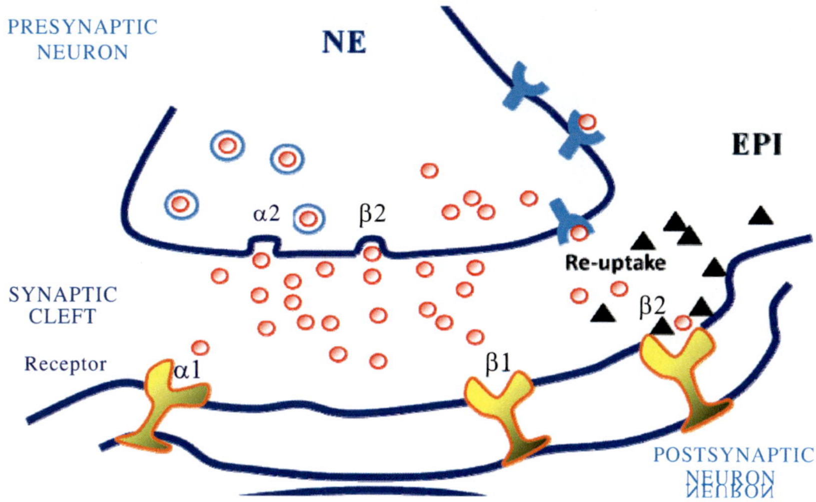

NE, norepinephrine ; EPI, epinephrine ▲

Figure 1. Schema of catecholamines and adrenoceptors at nerve endings.

There is evidence that epinephrine may be released as a co-transmitter from sympathetic nerves of normotensive and hypertensive subjects. [31, 32] There exists data which suggests that epinephrine is synthesized *in situ* in sympathetic nerve endings, which is induced by chronic mental stress exposure [33-35]. Interestingly, some patients with psychological disorders (*i.e.* major depression, panic disorder), who are at higher risk of development of cardiovascular disease, have extraordinarily higher sympathetic nerve activity compared to healthy controls [36-38]. Whether there exists a relationship between elevated norepinephrine and epinephrine secretion in these patient groups remains unknown.

The purpose of this article is to provide a summary of current findings on the relationship between epinephrine and blood pressure levels (hypertension). The contribution of epinephrine to the onset or development of hypertension including the "epinephrine hypothesis" will be explored through a review of available literature, matched against our own either published or unpublished findings.

Epinephrine Synthesis and Metabolism

Epinephrine is a catecholamine and is synthesized from tyrosine in sympathetic nerve terminals and in the adrenal gland (Figure 1). The first step, which is rate limiting, is the hydroxylation of tyrosine to form 3,4-dihydeoxyphenylalanine (DOPA). Epinephrine is formed by the methylation of norepinephrine by a transmethylase that utilizes S-adenosylmethionine. Catecholamine neurotransmitters are quickly inactivated by methylation of the 3-hydroxy group of the catechol ring (Figure 2-A). This reaction is catalyzed by catechol-O-methyltransferase, which uses S-adenosylmethionine as the methyl donor. Alternatively, these neurotransmitters can be inactivated by oxidative removal of their amino group by monoamine oxidase (Figure 2-B). Catecholamines may also be inactivated by conjugation of their phenolic hydroxy group with sulfate or glucuromide; the reaction occurs mainly in the liver, gut, and red blood cells. Catecholamines and metabolites are excreted in the urine. Normally, the proportions in urine of catecholamines and metabolites are approximately 50% metanephrine, 35% VMA, 10% conjugated catecholamines and other metabolites, and <5% free catecholamines.

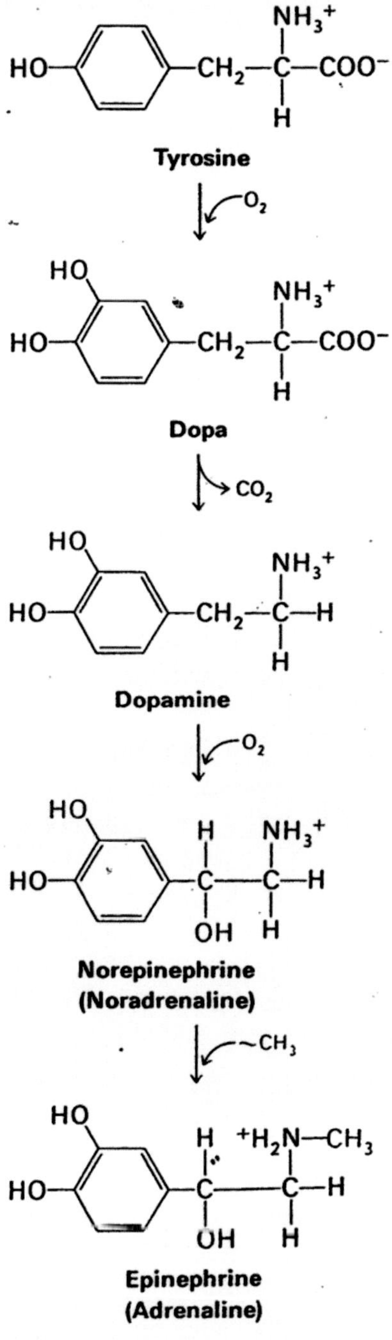

Figure 2 (A). Pathway for the synthesis of catecholamine neurotransmitter.

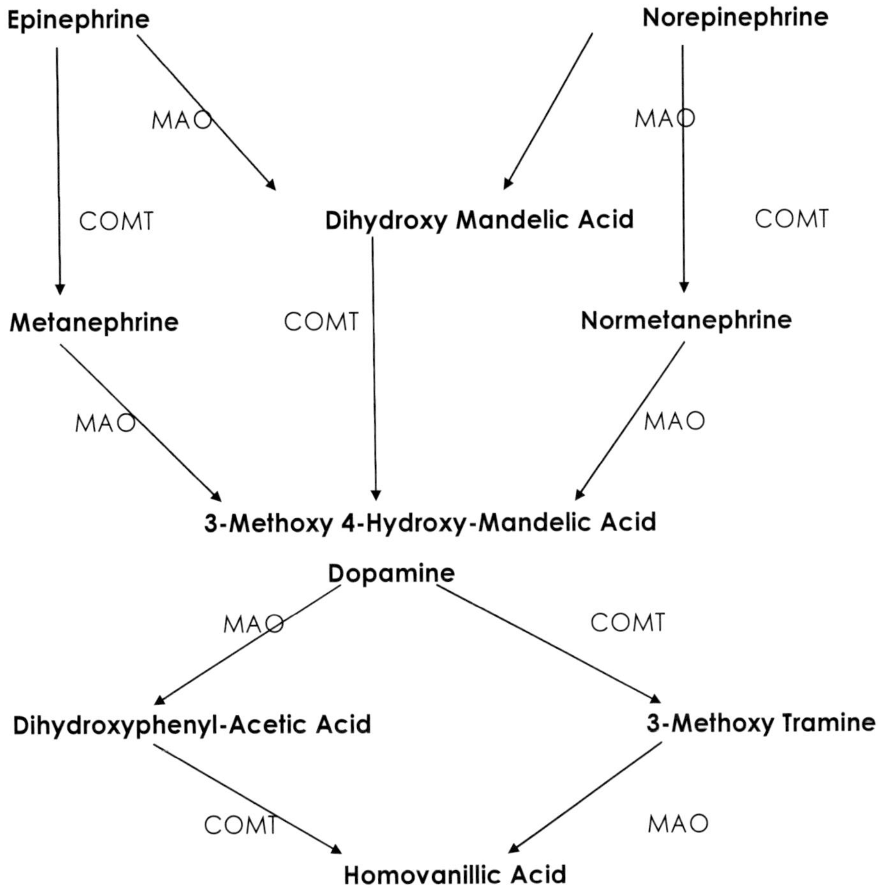

Figure 2 (B). Pathway for the metabolism of catecholamine neurotransmitter.

Epinephrine Secreted from Adrenal Medulla

The adrenal medulla is a specialized part of the sympathetic nervous system. It secretes catecholamines, especially epinephrine. The medullar of the adrenal glands in healthy humans contains 80% of epinephrine and 20% of norepinephrine. The sympathetic nervous system typically secretes norepinephrine as a local neurotransmitter directly in target organs. In comparison, the adrenal medulla is important for its secretion of epinephrine into the general circulation for widespread distribution and effect. Although, the adrenal medulla is not critically necessary for survival, its secretion of epinephrine and other compounds helps maintain the body homeostasis during stress. Investigations of the adrenal medulla and the sympathetic nervous system led to the discovery of different catecholamine receptors (see next section "Adrenoceptors subtypes") and the production of a wide variety of sympathetic agonists and antagonists with diverse clinical applications.

Adrenoceptors Subtypes and Function

The adrenoceptors (or adrenergic receptors) are a class of G protein-coupled receptor which specify bind their endogenous legends, the catecholamines (epinephrine and norepinephrine). Many tissues possess these receptors, and the binding of an agonist generally elicits a "typical" sympathetic response (*i.e.* the fight-or-flight response). For example, when catecholamines bind to adrenoceptors, the heart rate increases and the pupils dilate, energy is expended, and blood flow diverted from organs to skeletal muscle. Those effects by sympathetic nervous system are through α- and β-adrenergic receptors.

Table 1. Comparisons of adrenergic receptor subtypes

Receptor type	Agonist potency	Action sites	Functions
α1-adrenoceptor	norepinephrine ≥ epinephrine >>> isoprenaline	blood vessels of skin, gastrointestinal, kidney	vasoconstriction
		ureter, uterus, urethral spincter, bronchioles	smooth muscle
		urinary bladder	contraction
		iris, blood vessels of erectile tissue	smooth muscle relaxation
		heart muscle	positive ionotropic effect
		salivary gland	increase in secretion
		adipose tissue, liver	glycogenolysis and gluconeogenesis
		sweat glands	increase in secretion
		kidneys	Na reabsorption
α2-adrenoceptor	epinephrine > norepinephrine >>> isoprenaline	pancreas	inhibition of insulin secretion induction of glucagon release
		gastrointestinal tract	contraction of sphincters
β1-adrenoceptor	isoprenaline > norepinephrine > epinephrine	heart	increase cardiac output
		kidneys (juxtaglomerular cells)	increase renin release
		adipose tissue	lypolis
β2-adrenoceptor	isoprenaline > epinephrine >> norepinephrine	bronchi	smooth muscle relaxation
		urinary sphincter, bladder wall	smooth muscle relaxation
		skeletal muscle	dilate arteries
		adipose tissue, liver	glycogenolysis and gluconeogenesis
		gastrointestinal tract	contraction of sphincters
		salivary glands	thickened secretions
		mast cells	inhibit histamine-release
		kidneys (juxtaglomerular cells)	increase renin release
β3-adrenoceptor	isoprenaline > norepinephrine = epinephrine	adipose tissue	enhancement of lipolysis

Table 2. Studies in humans showing relationship between epinephrine and hypertension

Authors [reference number]	Year	Subjects	Results
Franco-Morselli R, et al. [27]	1977	NT vs. HT	Plasma EPI was higher in HT than in NT, but NE was similar between HT and NT.
Masuo K, et al. [13]	1983	NT vs. HT	Plasma EPI was similar between NT and HT under 3 different sodium balance in the supine and upright position,, but NE was higher in HT than in NT.
Goldstein DS, et al. [12]	1984	NT and HT	Plasma EPI was independent of age and NE in both NT and HT, while NE correlated with age in NT (but not in HT)
Masuo K, et al. [14]	1984	NT and EHT	Plasma EPI did not correlate with age in both NT and HT, while NE correlated with age in NT.
Goldstein DS, et al. [42]	1989	NT vs. EHT	HT had greater increases in EPI to mental stress, but EPI at rest was similar between NT and EHT.
Fujita T, et al [41]	1989	BHT vs. NT	Young BHT had higher plasma EPI than NT.
Perini C, et al. [46]	1990	BHT, FH+ vs. FH-	BHT with FH+ had higher plasma EPI at rest.
Jacobs MC, et al. [54]	1995	EHT	Chronic α1-adrenergic blocker did not change plasma EPI, total-body EPI spillover, or EPI clearance.
Manuck SB, et al. [49]	1996	NT, FH+ vs. FH-	Plasma or urinary EPI was similar between FH+ and FH-.
Jacobs MC, et al. [25]	1997	mild EHT	Adrenomedullary secretion of EPI was higher in mild EHT.
Yoshiuchi K, et al. [35]	1997	EHT	Mental stress increased plasma EPI levels. Changes in EPI correlated with changes in BP and changes in cardiac output, but did not NE.
Stein MC, et al. [5]	1997	NT vs. BHT	Short-term local infusion of EPI did not facilitate forearm NE spillover.
Grassi G. [11]	1998	NT vs. HT	Plasma EPI was similar between NT and HT, but NE was higher in HT.
Lee ZS, et al. [55]	2001	population study (Chinese)	Urinary EPI was related to BP levels through BMI.
Reims HM, et al. [34]	2004	BHT vs. NT,	Lean BHT had greater responses in EPI to mental stress.
Masuo K, et al. [52, 53]	2005, 2006	nonobese, NT	Plasma EPI was not related with β2-adrenoceptor polymorphism
Flaa A, et al. [56]	2006	NT and HT	BP levels at rest predicted increases in plasma EPI, NE and BP elevation during mental stress.

EPI, epinephrine; NE, norepinephrine; BP, blood pressure; BMI, body mass index; NT, normotensive subjects; HT, hypertensive patients; BHT, patients with borderline hypertension; EHT, patients with essential hypertension; FH+, a positive family history of hypertension; FH-, a negative family history of hypertension.

There are several types of adrenergic receptors, but there are two main groups: α-adrenoceptors (α1- and α2-adrenoceptors) and β-adrenoceptors (β1-, β2-, and β3-adrenoceptors). Table 1 summaries the distributions and functions of the α1-, α2-, β1-, β2-, and β3-adrenoceptors. [28, 39] The α-receptors bind norepinephrine and epinephrine, though norepinephrine has higher affinity. Phenylephrine is a selective agonist of the α-adrenoceptors (both α1- and α2-receptors), thus phenylephrine is usually used to investigate the α-adrenoceptors function. β-adrenoceptors are linked to G proteins, which are linked to adenyl cyclase. β-adrenoceptor agonists cause the intracellular elevation of the second messenger cyclic AMP. Downstream effects of cyclic AMP include cyclic AMP dependent protein kinase (PKA), which mediates the intracellular events following hormone binding.

Role of Epinephrine or Sympathetic Nervous Activation in Hypertension: Clinical and Epidemiological Studies (Table 2)

Thirty years ago Franco-Morselli *et al.* [27] reported that epinephrine is more important in hypertension than norepinephrine. Several investigators have also observed that essential hypertensive patients or borderline hypertensive patients have higher plasma epinephrine levels [40, 41], higher epinephrine secretion from the adrenal medulla [25] and enhanced cardiovascular responses to physical or psychological stress [34, 35, 42]. Sherwood *et al.* [43] found that borderline hypertensive patients exhibit pressor hyperactivity during mental and physiological stress, with the response being associated with greater increases in plasma epinephrine. Recently, Reims *et al.* [34] reported that lean borderline hypertensive patients have enhanced response in plasma epinephrine to mental stress or to hyperinsulinemic glucose clamp. They concluded that adrenal medullary activation plays an important role in blood pressure elevation in lean borderline hypertension. Interestingly, Jacobs *et al.* [25] have reported that hypertensive patients have higher arterial epinephrine concentrations and whole-body epinephrine spillover, but norepinephrine spillover or norepinephrine concentrations are normal. (Figure 3) In contrast, Grassi [11] and Masuo *et al.* [13, 14, 17, 19] have observed that hypertensive patients or subjects who subsequently develop blood pressure elevation in the future have higher levels of plasma norepinephrine, but similar levels of epinephrine. (Figure 4, Figure 5)

In 1983 Goldstein [44] performed a meta-analysis of 78 comparative studies of plasma catecholamines, but mainly focusing on norepinephrine, in normotensive and essential hypertensive subjects. Most reported higher norepinephrine levels in the hypertensive patients, although only about 40% of the studies were positive with statistically significant hypertensive-normotensive differences. Although there was dramatic variability in catecholamine values within and across studies, they concluded that virtually all studies of catecholamines (norepinephrine + epinephrine) in young, consistently hypertensive patients were positive. [44] Importantly, there are a number of confounding variables that need to be considered when examining the relationships between epinephrine and hypertension. These include, but are not limited to, ethnicity [45], age [10, 14], gender [24], posture and mental [13, 38, 46] or physical stress [47], severity of hypertension [14, 19, 46], sodium intake states [13, 14, 48] or genetic background of hypertension (family history of hypertension) [22, 46, 49].

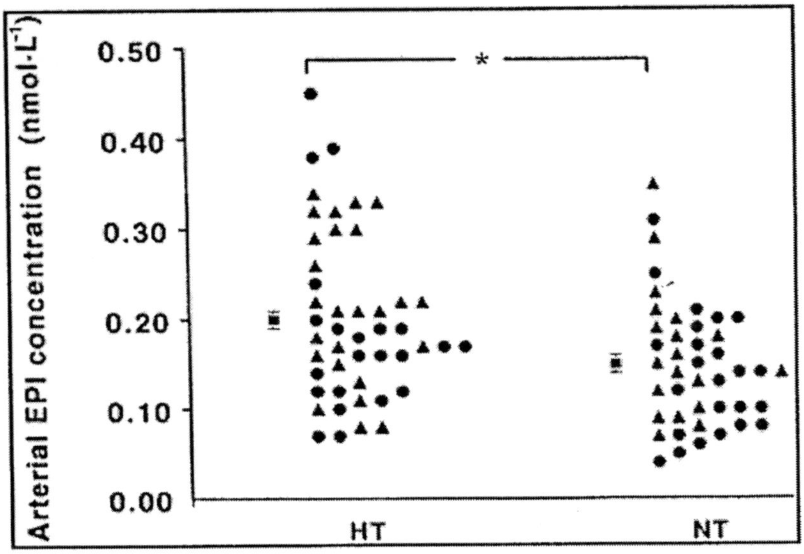

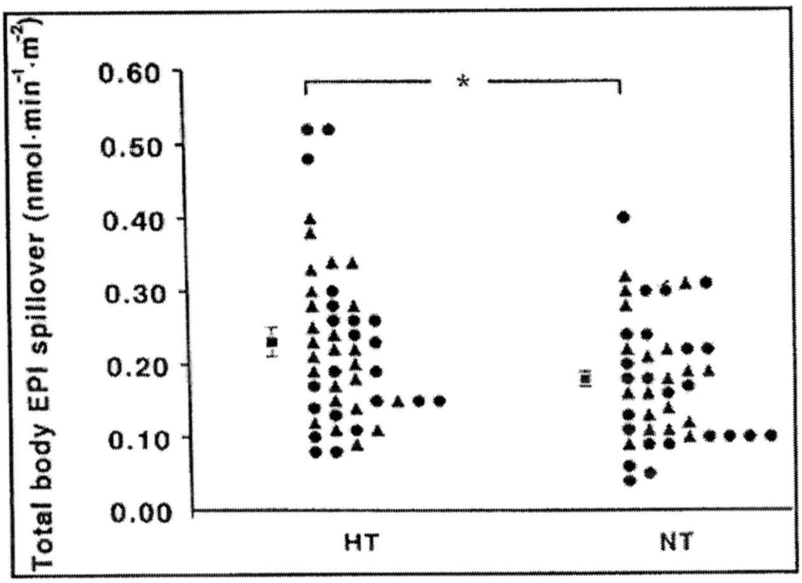

*P<0.05 versus normotensive subjects. EPI, epinephrine; HT, mild essential hypertensive patients (n=47); NT, normotensive subjects (n=43). ▲ male; • female. *Jacobs MC, et al. Hypertension. 1997. [25]*

Figure 3. Arterial plasma epinephrine concentration and whole-body epinephrine spillover were significantly higher in hypertensive patients.

Masuo *et al.* [13] observed that plasma epinephrine levels were similar between young, age-matched normotensive and mild hypertensive subjects under 3 different levels of sodium balance (low, regular, and high sodium intakes). These investigations were performed in both the supine and upright positions (Figure 5). Plasma epinephrine was raised considerably in the upright position in both normotensive and hypertensive patients. The effect was most prominent especially in the low sodium intake. [13] Plasma norepinephrine concentrations increase with age in normotensive subjects, whereas plasma epinephrine concentrations are independent of age and norepinephrine levels (Figure 6). [10, 14] Regarding the family history of hypertension, Masuo *et al.* [22] compared plasma epinephrine and norepinephrine levels in normotensive subjects with and without a positive family history of hypertension. Plasma norepinephrine levels were significantly higher in subjects who had a strong family history of hypertension compared to those without a family history of hypertension, but plasma epinephrine levels were similar between those with and without a positive family history of hypertension (unpublished data). Plasma norepinephrine, but not plasma epinephrine levels, could predict future blood pressure elevation [15] and weight gain [51] in longitudinal studies of 10 years. The series of studies conducted by Masuo *et al.* demonstrates that epinephrine does not play an important role in the onset and the maintenance of hypertension. [13-15, 17-19, 51-53]

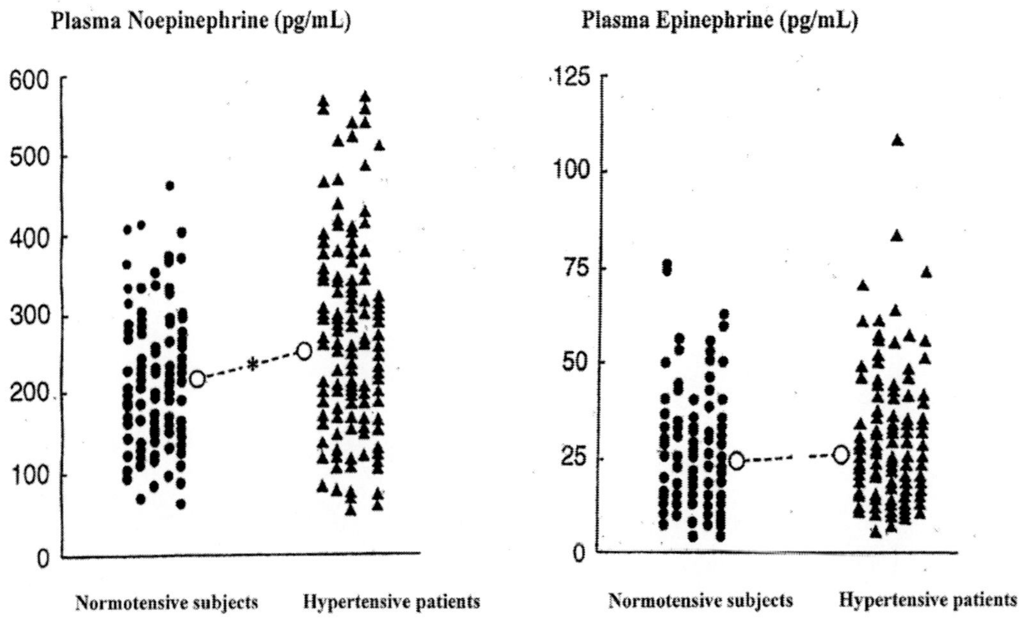

*P<0.05 versus normotensive subjects. Plasma norepinephrine levels were significantly higher in hypertensive patients compared to normotensive subjects, but plasma epinephrine levels were similar in the study consisting of 131 normotensive and 172 hypertensive subjects. *Grassi G, et al. J Hypertens. 1998. [11]*

Figure 4. Plasma epinephrine levels were similar between normatensive and hypertensive subjects.

The effects of the β2-adrenoceptor polymorphisms (Arg16Gly, Gln27Glu) or β3-adrenoceptor polymorphisms (Trp64Arg) on hypertension development have demonstrated a genetic component in the etiology of elevated blood pressure. In a longitudinal study over a 5-year period in 160 young, nonobese, normotensive men, Masuo and colleagues showed that the Gly16 allele of the Arg16Gly, β2-adrenoceptor polymorphism, was related to significant blood pressure elevation (>10% from the entry period). [52, 53] The subjects carrying the Gly16 allele of Arg16Gly had significantly higher plasma norepinephrine concentrations, but plasma epinephrine concentrations were similar. (Figure 7) This observation suggests that epinephrine acts at the β2-adrenoceptors, but the β2-adrenoceptor does not regulate epinephrine secretion.

Plasma epinephrine levels

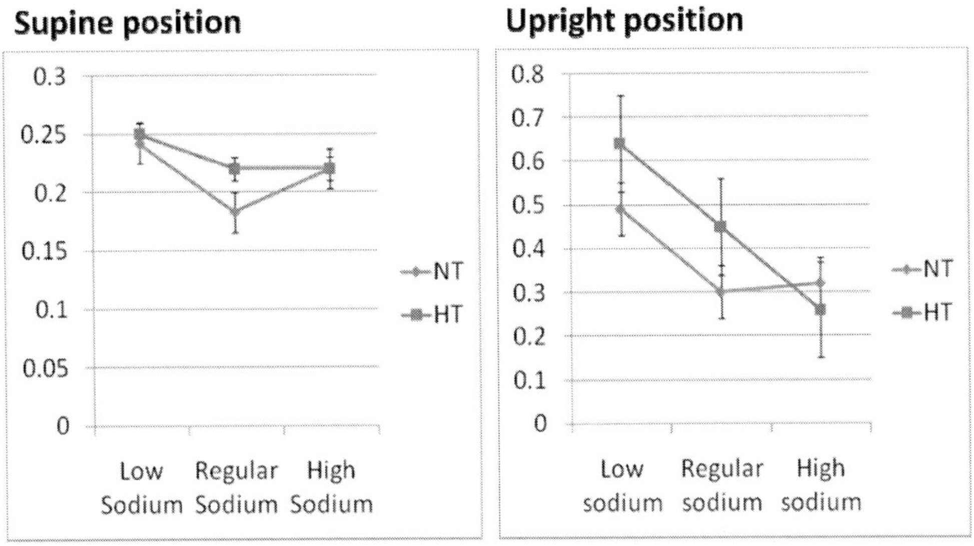

Plasma norepinephrine levels

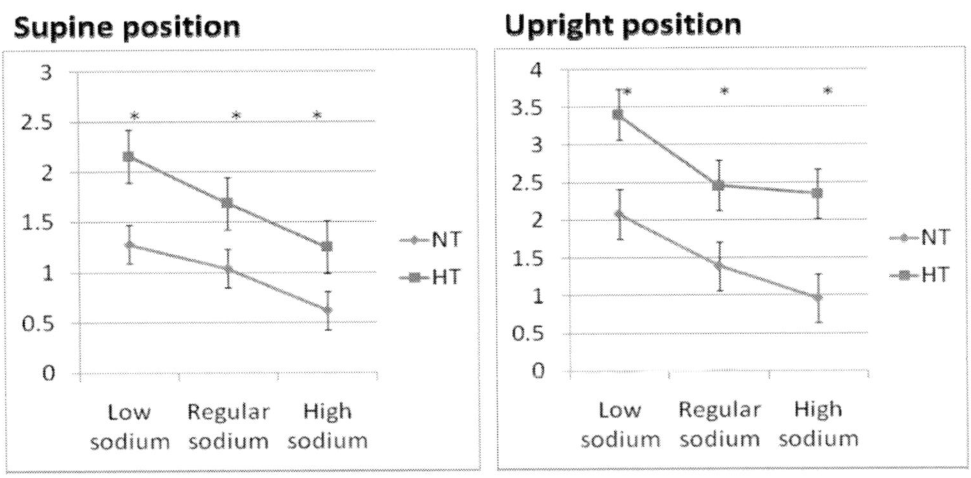

NT, normotensive subjects; HT, hypertensive patients. *P<0.05 versus normotensive subjects. Twenty-four normotensive and 38 hypertensive subjects were measured plasma epinephrine and norepinephrine after 5 days on each sodium balance. Plasma norepinephrine levels were higher in hypertensive patients compared to normotensive subjects throughout the study, but plasma epinephrine levels were similar to those in normotensive subjects. *Masuo K, et al. Hypertension. 1983. [13]*

Figure 5. Comparisons of plasma epinephrine and norepinephrine levels between normotensive and hypertensive subjects under three sodium balance (low, regular, and high sodium intakes) in supine position and upright position.

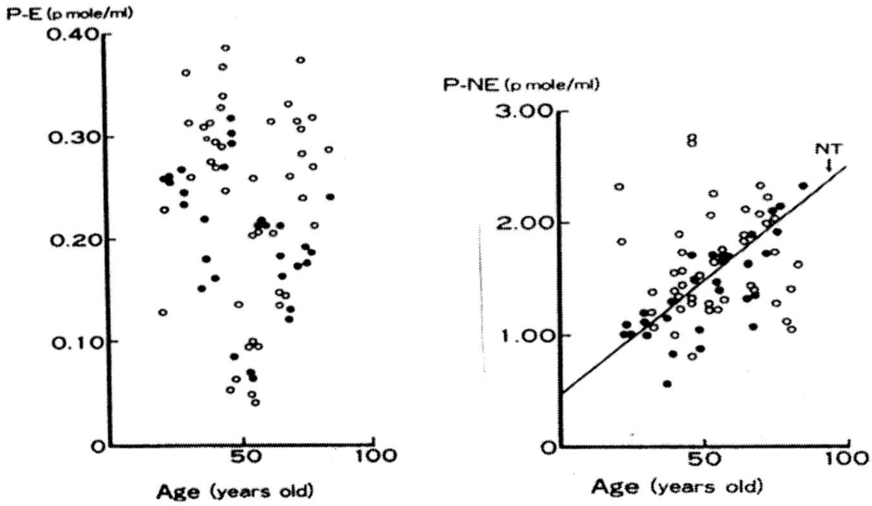

P-E, plasma epinephrine concentration; P-NE, plasma norepinephrine concentration. NT, normotensive subjects (•); hypertensive patients (o). Thirty normotensive subjects and 44 hypertensive subjects with a wide range of age were measured plasma epinephrine and norepinephrine levels. Plasma norepinephrine levels increased with age in normotensive subjects, whereas plasma epinephrine levels was not related with age. *Masuo K, et al. Hypertension. 1984. [14]*

Figure 6. Plasma epinephrine does not increase with age in normotensive subjects, but plasma norepinephrine increased with age.

Plasma norepinephrine levels are higher in subjects carrying the Gly16 allele, but plasma epinephrine levels are similar.

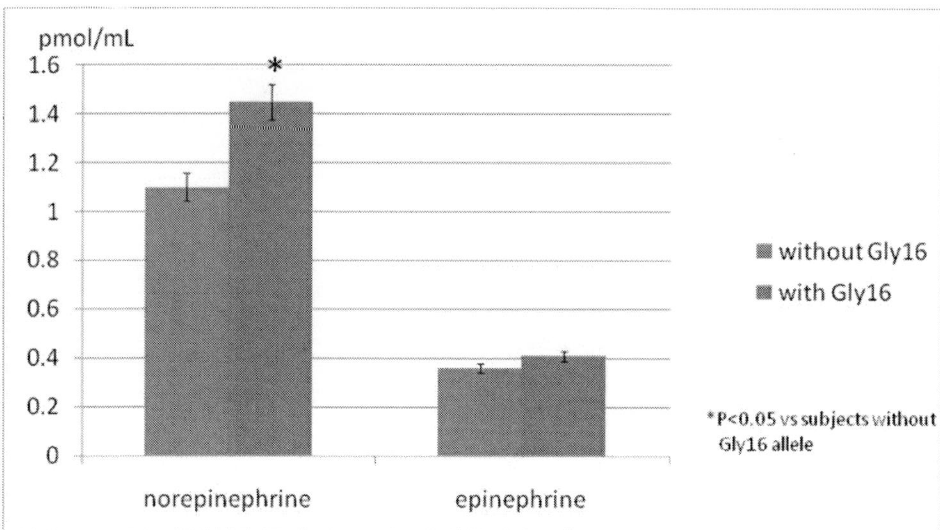

Plasma norepinephrine and epinephrine were measured in 160 young, nonobese, normotensive subjects consisting of 115 subjects carrying the Gly16 allele and 45 without the Gly16 allele of Arg16Gly. Plasma norepinephrine levels were significantly higher in subjects carrying the Gly16 allele, but plasma epinephrine levels were similar. *Masuo K, et al. Circulation. 2005. [52]*

Figure 7. Plasma norepinephrine and epinephrine levels according to the β2-adrenoceptor polymorphism (Arg16Gly)

Role of Epinephrine in Hypertension: Animal Studies (Table 3)

Many results, but not all, from animal studies show strong relationships between epinephrine or sympatho-adrenomedullary function and hypertension. Using the adrenal demedullation technique, Borkowski *et al.* [29] reported that epinephrine from the adrenal medulla played a major role in hypertension development and vascular reactivity in young spontaneously hypertensive rats. Several other investigators using pharmacological tools [48, 50] have also demonstrated that epinephrine and sympatho-adrenomedullary function play an important role in hypertension. However, several studies have shown no relationship between epinephrine and hypertension in animal models [28, 30]. Important studies are summarized in table 3. (Table 3)

Table 3. Studies in animal models showing relationship between epinephrine and hypertension

Authors [reference number]	Year	Animal	Results
Black J, et al. [57]	1981	DOCA-salt hypertensive rats	Central epinephrine regulated peripheral sympatho-adrenomedullary and barosensitivity.
Szemeredi K, et al. [58]	1988	SHR vs. WKY rats	In juvenile SHR sympatho-adrenomedullary activity was elevated compared to WKY or matured SHR. (positive data)
Tarizzo VI, et al. [59]	1989	pithed rats with adrenal medullarectomy	In adrenal demedullated rats, BP response to stimulation was attenuated, but during exogenous EPI infusion, BP response was enhanced. (positive data)
Turkkan JS, et al. [48]	1991	baboons	Sodium loading and stress increased BP, but urinary NE and EPI did not change. (sodium balance, negative data)
Borkowski KR. [29]	1991	young SHR with adrenal medullarectomy	Young adrenal demedullated SHR had significant lower plasma EPI, but BP elevation was attenuated. (negative data)
Lo M, et al. [30]	1991	Lyon-hypertensive or normotensive with adrenal medullarectomy	Adrenal demedullation caused EPI production, but BP difference between NT and HT was not different from those before demedullation. (negative data)
Kaufman LN, et al. [60]	1993	SD rats with adrenal medullectomy	High fat and glucose diet cause obesity and BP elevation, but no increases in urinary EPI excretion in adrenal demedullated rats. (obesity –related hypertension, negative data)
Jablonckis LT, et al. [28]	1994	SD or SHR-SP with adrenal medullarectomy	SHR-SP demedullated rats had significant reduction in EPI in plasma and adrenal, but BP was higher than control rats. (negative data)

Table 3. (Continued)

Authors [reference number]	Year	Animal	Results
Lange DL, et al. [24]	1998	DOCA-salt rats	Male DOCA-salt rats had significantly higher catecholamine content in the adrenal medulla than female DOCA-salt rats. (gender difference)
Kanayama K, et al. [47]	1999	WKY rats	WKY rats in the cold stress had significantly higher plasma EPI, NE and BP compare to those in room temperature. (positive data)
Lange DL, et al. [61]	2000	DOCA-salt hypertensive rats	Conscious DOCA-salt rats had higher levels of BP compared to control rats, but NE and EPI did not differ between control rats and DOCA-salt hypertensive rats. (negative data)

EPI, epinephrine; NE, norepinephrine; BP, blood pressure; SHR, spontaneously hypertensive rats; SHR-SP, spontaneously hypertensive stroke prone rats; WKY, Wister-Kyoto rats; SD rats, Sprague-Dawley rats; DOCA-salt rats, deoxycorticosterone acetate and salt rats.

Epinephrine Hypothesis

The fundamentals of the "epinephrine hypothesis" are quite simple and, in effect rest on the contention that: epinephrine could be taken up into postgnaglionic sympathetic nerves and be released as a co-transmitter with norepinephrine (NE) (1-3, 62-64). When released, epinephrine augments the simultaneous discharge of endogenous norepinephrine. Thus, the facilitated release of norepinephrine may occur after exogeneous administration of epinephrine (3, 5) or following sympatho-adrenomedullary stimulation. Thus, it is feasible that epinephrine could be closely linked to neurogenic vasoconstriction (blood pressure elevation, hypertension).

Relevant studies of the "epinephrine hypothesis" were searched using: (1) electronic search of PubMed (1990 to December 2007, NCBI interface) published in the English language, and (2) searching the reference lists of all included articles in order to ensure that all relevant material was obtained. Only 3 articles were found from PubMed. (1, 40, 65)

Several studies have reported that epinephrine can augment neurogenic vasoconstriction. Nezu *et al.* [31] studied the effects of endogenous epinephrine released by glucagon injection, and exogeneous epinephrine infusion on plasma norepinephrine and cardiovascular responses in patients with essential hypertension and in age-matched normotensive subjects. Elevation of endogenous epinephrine induced by glucagon injection caused significant elevation of plasma norepinephrine. An intravenous infusion of exogenous epinephrine caused a significant elevation of plasma norepinephrine and blood pressure. Thus, they concluded that plasma epinephrine could act physiologically as a sustained stimulator of pre-synaptic β-adrenoceptors, which leads to enhanced norepinephrine release from peripheral sympathetic nerve terminals and an elevation of blood pressure in humans. Majewski *et al.* [1-3] observed larger vasoconstrictor response in the forearm artery and norepinephrine elevation after epinephrine infusion compared to those before the epinephrine infusion. Floras *et al.*, in 23 healthy volunteers, examined whether epinephrine facilitates neurogenic vasoconstriction in humans [32]. They observed during 30 minutes after brachial intra-arterial epinephrine infusion, lower body negative pressure (LBNP) elicited a larger forearm vasoconstrictor response than before the epinephrine infusion. Their results are consistent with the "epinephrine hypothesis'. The "epinephrine hypothesis" helps to explain how excessive adreno-medullary hormonal system activity can contribute to the development of essential hypertension by augmenting sympatho-neural norepinephrine release. [1-4]

In contrast, adrenalectomized humans have normal vascular and plasma norepinephrine responses to various stimulations, which also argue against the epinephrine effects as neurogenic vasoconstriction. [6] Thompson *et al.* [65] and Goldstein *et al.* [66] observed that intra-arterial or intra-venous epinephrine did not augment cardiac norepinephrine spillover or forearm norepinephrine spillover in humans. Stein *et al.* [5] reported that forearm norepinephrine spillover was not augmented after intra-arterial epinephrine infusion at a brachial artery even at the same infusion dose used in Floras' previous study [32], where they observed strong augmentation of forearm norepinephrine spillover. Intra-arterial infusion of isoproterenol to stimulate forearm norepinephrine spillover showed no delayed facilitator effects of intra-arterial isoproterenol. They concluded that the short-term local infusion of epinephrine does not have a delayed facilitatory effect on forearm norepinephrine spillover in normotensive and borderline hypertensive subjects. Interestingly, Goldstein *et al.* [67] examined very carefully in 40 healthy, nonobese volunteers with the same design using the same procedure (the same dose of epinephrine infusion of a physiologically active dose; the same infusion site (brachial artery); using the same stimulation (LBNP); norepinephrine measurement method (radioisotope dilution technique)) to that of the previous study conducted by Floras [32]. However, loading of forearm sympathetic terminals with epinephrine did not augment subsequent neurogenic vasoconstriction, norepinephrine release, arterio-venous increments in plasma norepinephrine levels or forearm norepinephrine spillover response in the human forearm in response to sympathetic stimulation. These results [6, 66, 67] are inconsistent with the "epinephrine hypothesis".

Floras [67] suggested that the discordant findings on the "epinephrine hypothesis" and expression of hypertension due to "the "epinephrine hypothesis" might be restricted to a specific epinephrine-sensitive subset of individuals with a genetic predisposition to high blood pressure. This is an interesting thought given that only genetic models of hypertensive rats have critical sensitivity to endogenous epinephrine.

Conclusion

The role of epinephrine on hypertension and the "epinephrine hypothesis" are discussed through a literature review including either published or unpublished data. Relevant studies of the sympathetic nervous system activity in relation to hypertension were investigated, however, not so many investigations have included epinephrine, although epinephrine is the most effective drug for treating cardiac shock or anaphylaxis and pheochromocytoma is known for its hypertension caused by very high epinephrine (and norepinephrine) secretion from the adrenal gland(s) or extra-adrenall chromaffin cells. Thus, the relationships between epinephrine and hypertension as represented in the "epinephrine hypothesis" are still controversial. Further studies are necessary to clarify the relationships of epinephrine with hypertension (cardiovascular disease) and to understand further the precise role of epinephrine on the cardiovascular system.

References

[1] Majewski H, Tung LH, Rand MJ. (1981) Hypertension through adrenaline activation of prejunctional beta-adrenoceptor. *Clin Exp Pharmacol Physiol.* 8: 463-468.

[2] Majewski H, Tung LH, Rand MJ. (1982) Adrenaline activation of prejunctional beta-adrenoceptors and hypertension. *J Cardiovasc Pharmacol.* 4: 99-106.

[3] Rand MJ, Majewski H. (1984) Adrenaline mediates a positive feedback loop in noradrenergic transmission: its possible role in development of hypertension. *Clin Exp Hypertens.* A6: 347-370.

[4] Floras JS, Sole MJ, Morris BL. (1990) Despiramine blocks augmented neurogenic vasoconstrictor responses to epinephrine. *Hypertension.* 15: 132-139.

[5] Stein CM, Nelson R, He HB, Wood M, Wood AJ. (1997) Norepinephrine release in the human forearm: effects of epinephrine. *Hypertension.* 30: 1078-1084.

[6] Lenders JW, Peters JH, Pieters GF, Wilemen JJ, Thien T. (1988) Hemodynamic reactivity to sympathoadrenal stimulation in adrenalectomized women. *J Clin Endocrinol Metab.* 67: 139-143.

[7] Stjarne L, Brundin J. (1975) Dual adrenoceptors mediated control of noradrenaline secretion from human vasoconstrictor nerves: facilitation by beta-receptors and ingibition by alpha-receptors. *Acta Physiol Scand.* 94: 139-141.

[8] Stjarne L, Brundin J. (1976) Beta2-adrenoceptor facilitatring noradrenaline secretion from human vasoconstristor nerves. *Acta Physiol Scand.* 97: 88-93.

[9] Dahlof C. (1981) Studies on beta-adrenoceptor mediatred facilitation of sympathetic neurotransmission. *Acta Physiol Scand Suppl.* 500: 1-147.

[10] Esler M, Lambert G, Kaye D, Rumantir M, Hastings J, Seals DR. (2002) Influence of ageing on the sympathetic nervous system and adrenal medulla at rest and during stress. *Biogerontology.* 3: 45-49.

[11] Grassi G. (1998) Role of the sympathetic nervous system in human hypertension. *J Hypertens.* 16: 1979-1987.

[12] Goldstein DS, Lake CR. (1984) Plasma norepinephrine and epinephrine levels in essential hypertension. *Fed Proc.* 43: 57-61.

[13] Masuo K, Ogihara T, Kumahara Y, Yamatodani A, Wada H. (1983) Plasma norepinephrine and dietary sodium intake in normal subjects and patients with essential hypertension. *Hypertension.* 5: 767-771.

[14] Masuo K, Ogihara T, Kumahara Y, Yamatodani A, Wada H. (1984) Increased plasma norepinephrine in young patients with essential hypertension under three sodium intakes. *Hypertension.* 6: 315-321.

[15] Masuo K, Mikami H, Ogihara T, Tuck ML. (2003) Serum uric acid and plasma norepinephrine concentrations predict subsequence weight gain and blood pressure elevation. *Hypertension.* 42: 474-480.

[16] Masuo K. (2002) Obesity-related hypertension: role of the sympathetic nervous system, insulin, and leptin. *Curr Hypertens Rep.* 4: 112-118.

[17] Masuo K, Mikami H, Itoh M, Ogihara T, Tuck ML. (2000) Sympathetic activity and body mass index contribute to blood pressure levels. *Hypertens Res.* 23: 303-310.

[18] Masuo K, Mikami H, Ogihara T, Tuck ML. (1997) Prevalence of hyperinsulinemia in young, nonobese Japanese men. *J Hypertens.* 25: 157-165.

[19] Masuo K, Mikami H, Ogihara T, Tuck ML. (1997) Sympathetic nerve hyperactivity precedes hyperinsulinemia and blood pressure elevation in a young, nonobese Japanese population. *Am J Hypertens.* 10: 77-83.

[20] Ward KD, Sparrow D, Landberg L, Young JB, Vokonas PS, Weiss ST. (1996) Influence of insulin, sympathetic nervous system activity, and obesity on blood pressure: the Normative Aging Study. *J Hypertens.* 14: 301-308.

[21] Esler M, Straznicky N, Eikelis N, Masuo K, Lambert G, Lambert E. (2006) Mechanisms of sympathetic activation in obesity-related hypertension. *Hypertension.* 48: 787-796.

[22] Masuo K, Mikami H, Ogihara T, Tuck ML. (1998) Familial hypertension, insulin, sympathetic activity, and blood pressure elevation. Hypertension. 32: 96-100.

[23] Tarizzo VI, Dahlof C. (1989) Adrenaline-induced enhancement of blood pressure response to sympathetic nerve stimulation in adrenal demedullated pithed rats. *Naunyn Schmiedebergs Arch Pharmacol.* 340: 144-150.

[24] Lange DL, Haywood JR, Hinojosa-Laborde C. (1998) Role of the adrenal medullae in male and female DOCA-salt hypertensive rats. *Hypertension.* 31(1 Pt 2): 403-408.

[25] Jacobs MC, Lenders JWM, Willemsen JJ, Thien T. (1997) Adrenomedullary secretion of epinephrine is increased in mild essential hypertension. *Hypertension.* 29: 1303-1308.

[26] Landsberg L. (1999) Role of sympathetic adrenal system in the pathogenesis of the insulin resistance syndrome. *Ann NY Acad Sci.* 892: 84-90.

[27] Franco-Morselli R, Elghozi JL, Joly E, Di Giuilio S, Meyer P. (1977) Increased plasma adrenaline concentrations in benign essential hypertension. *Br Med J.* 2: 1251-1254.

[28] Jablonskis LT, Howe PR. (1994) Lack of influence of circulating adrenaline on blood pressure in normotensive and hypertensive rats. *Blood Press.* 3: 112-119.

[29] Borkowski KR. (1991) Effect of adrenal demedullation and adrenaline on hypertension development and vascular reactivity in young spontaneous hypertensive rats. *J Auton Pharmacol.* 11: 1-14.

[30] Lo M, Julien C, Barres C, Boomsma F, Cerutti C, Vincent M, Sassard J. (1991) Blood pressure maintenance in hypertensive sympathectomised rats. Adrenal medullary catecholamines. *Am J Physiol.* 261: R10-45-R1051.

[31] Nezu M, Miura Y, Adachi M, Adachi M, Kimura S, Toriyabe S, Ishizuka Y, Ohashi H, Sugawara T, Takahashi M. (1985) The effects of epinephrine on norepinephrine release in essential hypertension. *Hypertension.* 7: 187-192.

[32] Floras JS, Aylward PE, Victor RG, Mark AL, Abboud FM. (1988) Epinephrine facilitates neurogenic vasoconstriction in humans. *J Clin Invest.* 81: 1265-1274.

[33] Esler M, Lux A, Jennings G, Hastings J, Socratous F, Lambert G. (2004) Rilmenidine sympatholytic activity preserves mental stress, orthostatic sympathetic responses and adrenaline secretion. *J Hypertens.* 22: 1529-1534.

[34] Reims HM, Fossum E, Heieggen A, Moan A, Eide I, Kjeldsen SE. (2004) Adrenal medullary overactivity in lean, borderline hypertensive young men. *Am J Hypertens.* 17: 611-618.

[35] Yoshiuchi K, Nomura S, Ando K, Ohtake T, Shimosawa T, Kumano H, Kubori T, Suematsu H, Fujita T. (1997) Hemodynamic and endocrine responsiveness to mental arithmetic task and mirror drawing test in patients with essential hypertension. *Am J Hypertens.* 10: 243-249.

[36] Barton DA, Dawood T, Lambert EA, Esler MD, Haikerwal D, Brenchley C, Socratous F, Kaye DM, Schlaich MP, Hickie I, Lambert GW. (2007) Sympathetic activity in major depressive disorder: identifying those at increased cardiac risk? *J Hypertens.* 25: 2117-2124.

[37] Alvarenga ME, Richards JC, Lambert G, Esler MD. (2006) Psychophysiological mechanisms in panic disorder: a correlative analysis of noradrenaline spillover, neuronal noradrenaline reuptake, power spectral analysis of heart rate variability, and psychological variables. *Psychosom Med.* 68: 8-16.

[38] Anderson EA, Sinkey CA, Mark AL. (1991) Mental stress increases sympathetic nerve activity during sustained baroreceptor stimulation in humans. *Hypertension.* 17 [suppl III]: III-43-III-49.

[39] Doda M. (1997) Role of different subtypes of adrenoceptors in pressor responses to catercholamines released from sympathetic nerve ending. *Brain Res Bull.* 42: 51-57.

[40] Buhler FR, Amann FW, Bolli P, Hulthen L, Kiowski W, Landmann R, Burgiser E. (1982) Elevated adrenaline and increased α-adrenoceptor-mediated vasoconstriction in essential hypertension. *J Cardiovasc Pharmacol.* 4: S134-S138.

[41] Fujita T, Noda H, Ito Y, Isaka M, Sato Y, Ogata E. (1989) Increased sympatho-adrenomedullary activity and left ventricular hypertrophy in young patients with borderline hypertension. *J Mol Cell Cardiol.* 21 (Suppl 5): 31-38.

[42] Goldstein DS, Eisenhofer G, Garty M, Sax FL, Keiser HR, Kopin IJ. (1989) Pharmacologic and tracer methods to study sympathetic function in primary hypertension. *Clin Exp Hypertens A.* 11 (Suppl 1): 173-189.

[43] Sherwood A, Hinderliter AL, Light KC. (1995) Physiological determinants of hyperreactivity to stress in borderline hypertension. *Hypertension.* 25: 384-392.

[44] Goldstein DS. (1983) Plasma catecholamines and essential hypertension. An analytical review. *Hypertension.* 5: 86-99.

[45] Carstensen E, Ramaiya K, Denver E, Mohamed-Ali V, Yudkin JS. (1995) The contribution of the sympatho-adrenomedullary system to the etiology of essential hypertension: A study using plasma and platelet catecholamine concentrations. *J Clin Endocrinol Metab.* 80: 455-460.

[46] Perini C, Muller FB, Rauchfleisch U, Battegay R, Buhler FR. (1990) Effects of psychological and physical covariates on plasma catecholamines in borderline

hypertensives and offspring of hypertensive patients. *Clin Exp Hypertens A.* 112: 137-150.

[47] Kanayama N, Khatun S, Belayet H, She L, Terao T. (1999) Chronic local cold stress to the soles induces hypertension in rats. *Am J Hypertens.* 12: 1124-1129.

[48] Turkkan JS, Goldstein DS. (1991) Stress and sodium hypertension in baboons: neuroendocrine and pharmacotherapeutic assessments. *J Hypertens.* 9: 969-975.

[49] Manuck SB, Polefrone JM, Terrell DF, Muldoon MF, Kasprowicz AL, Waldstein SR, Jennings RJ, Malkoff SB, Marsland A, Graham RE. (1996) Absemce of enhanced sympathoadrenal activity and behaviourally evoked cardiovascular reactivity among offspring of hypertensives. *Am J Hypertens.*9: 248-255.

[50] Chu CP, Qiu DL, Kato K, Kunitake T, Watanabe S, Yu NS, Nakazato M, Kannan H. (2004) Central stresscopin modulates cardiovascular function through the adrenal medulla in conscious rats. *Regul Pept.* 119: 53-59.

[51] Masuo K, Mikami H, Ogihara T, Tuck ML. (2000) Weight gain-induced blood pressure elevation. *Hypertension.* 35: 1135-1140.

[52] Masuo K, Katsuya T, Fu Y, Rakugi H, Ogihara T, Tuck ML. (2005) Beta2- and beta3-adrenergic receptor polymorphisms are related to the onset of weight gain and blood pressure elevation over 5 years. *Circulation.* 111: 3429-3434.

[53] Kawaguchi H, Masuo K, Katsuya T, Sugimoto K, Rakugi H, Ogihara T, Tuck ML. (2006) Beta2- and beta3-adrenoceptor polymorphisms relate to subsequent weight gain and blood pressure elevation in obese normotensive individuals. *Hypertens Res.* 29: 951-959.

[54] Jacobs MC, Lenders JW, Willemsen JJ, Thien T. (1995) Chronic alpha-1adrenergic blockade increases sympathoneural but not adreno-medullary activity in patients with essential hypertension. *J Hypertens.* 13: 1837-1841.

[55] Lee ZS, Critchley JA, Tomlinson B, Young RP, Thomas GN, Cockram CS, Chan TY, Chan JC. (2001) Urinary epinephrine and norepinephrine interrelations with obesity, insulin, and the metabolic syndrome in HongKong Chinese. *Metabolism.* 50: 135-143.

[56] Flaa A, Mundal HH, Eide I, Kjeldsen S, Rostrup M. (2006) Sympathetic activity and cardiovascular risk factors in young men in the low, normal, and high blood pressure ranges. *Hypertension.* 47: 396-402.

[57] Black J, Waeber B, Bresnahan MR, Gavras I, Gavras H. (1981) Blood pressure response to central and/or peripheral inhibition of phenylethanolamine N-methyltransferase in normotensive and hypertensive rats. *Circ Res.* 49: 518-524.

[58] Szemerdi K, Bagdy G, Stull R, Keiser HR, Kopin IJ, Goldstein DS. (1988) Sympathoadrenomedullary hyper-sensitiveness to yohimbine in juvenile spontaneous hypertensive rats. *Life Sci.* 43: 1063-1068.

[59] Tarizzo VI, Dahlof C. (1989) Adrenaline-induced enhancement of blood pressure response to sympathetic nerve stimulation in adrenal demedullated pithed rats. *Naunyn Schmiedebergs Arch Pharmacol.* 340: 144-150.

[60] Kaufman LN, Li HY, Peterson MM, Gilardy AK. (1993) Adrenal medulla as a mediator of diet-induced hypertension. *Am J Physiol.* 265 (1 Pt 2): R1-R6.

[61] Lange DL, Haywood JR, Hinojosa-Laborde C. (2000) Endothelin enhances and inhibits adrenal catecholamine release in deoxycorticosterone acetate-salt hypertensive rats. *Hypertension.* 35: 385-390.

[62] Quinn P, Borkowski KR, Collis MG. (1984) Epinephrine enhances neurogenic vasoconstriction in the rat perfused kidney. *Hypertension.* 7: 47-52.

[63] Dahlof C, Ljung B, Ablad B. (1978) Increased noradrenaline release in rat portal vein during sympathetic nerve stimulation due to activation of presynaptic beta-adrenoceptord by noradrenaline and adrenaline. *Eur J Pharmacol.* 50: 75-68.

[64] Rosell S, Axelrod J, Kopin IJ. (1964) Release of tritiated epinephrine following sympathetic nerve stimulation. *Nature.* 201: 301.

[65] Thompson JM, Sallin BG, Lambert GW, Jennings GL, Esler MD. (1998) Human muscle sympathetic activity and cardiac catecholamine spillover: no support for augmented sympathetic noradrenaline release by adrenaline co-transmission. *Clin Sci.* 94: 383-393.

[66] Goldstein DS, Golezynska A, Stuhlmuller J, Holmes C, Rea RF, Grossman E, Lenders J. (1999) A test of the 'epinephrine hypothesis" in human. *Hypertension.* 33: 36-43.

[67] Floras JS. (1992) Epinephrine and the genesis of hypertension. *Hypertension.* 19: 1-18.

In: Research Progress on Epinephrine ISBN: 978-1-60456-443-3
Editors: A. G. Lawson and R. I. Gorman, pp.115-127

Chapter VI

Pontine and Cerebellar Differential Norepinephrinergic Response after Cortical Ablation and Fe2Cl-induced Cortical Injury

***Rigoberto Gonzalez-Pina*[1,*], *Paloma DelaGarza-Montano*, *and Alfonso Alfaro-Rodriguez*[2]**

[1]Laboratorio de Neuroplasticidad, Instituto Nacional de Rehabilitacion, SSA
[2]Laboratorio de Neuroquimica. Instituto Nacional de Rehabilitacion, SSA

Abstract

It has been discussed that acute and slow-growing lesions involve different patterns of reorganization. Regarding the anatomical relationships between the motor cortex, the pons, and the cerebellum, we evaluated the effects of an acute lesion (cortical ablation) and a Fe2Cl-induced slow-growing lesion in order to study their effects on the pontine and cerebellar norepinephrine (NE) contents, since this neurotransmitter has been involved in the recovery of the lost functions.

Sixty-five male wistar rats (280-320 g) were allocated into six groups: sham-operated A (SA; n=11), sham-operated B (SB), injured by cortical ablation (CA), injured by cortical ablation and recovering (CAR), injured by Fe2Cl intraparenchimal injection in the motor cortex (Fe), and injured by the same procedure and recovering (FeR). Their footprints were obtained 24 hours before the surgery as a basal record. Then, 35 rats were operated upon and the right hindlimb motor area (MCx) was aspirated in the CA (N=6) and CAR (n=12) groups, while all the procedures without aspiration were performed in the SA (n=11) group. Then, the footprints were recorded every 6 hours for

* Corresponding author: Calz. Mexico-Xochimilco 289 Col. Arenal de Guadalupe Deleg. Tlalpan. C.P. 14389 Mexico City MEXICO tels. 52 55 59991000 ext. 19201 and 19214. e-mail: higgo65@ salud.gob.mx

48 hours. In the remaining subjects, a cannula directed to the MCx was surgically placed in the SB (n=16), Fe (n=5), and FeR (n=16) groups. Thus, artificial cerebrospinal fluid (CSF, 5μl) was injected in free-moving conditions in the SB animals, while CSF containing Fe2Cl (50 mM) was injected into the Fe and FeR groups. Footprints were recorded for 15 days. At the end of the recordings periods, the rats were sacrificed by decapitation and the left and right sides of the pons and cerebella were removed. NE contents were analyzed by HPLC, and the remaining encephallus was used in order to delimitate the respective lesions. Comparisons were performed using the Mann-Withney U test (p=0.05).

Results showed that recovery in ablated animals was faster than in Fe2Cl injured rats. We also observed a pontine NE increase in CA animals and a NE decrease in Fe rats, turning to normal levels in recovering rats. Cerebellar NE was unaltered in CA group, decreased in Fe animals and unaltered in FeR animals.

These results demonstrate that the NEergic mechanisms involved in the recovery after brain injury depends on the kind of the lesion. This suggests the need to evaluate the nature of the injury in order to develop clinical strategies in the treatment in humans.

Introduction

Studies focused on the effects of either the slow-growing or acute lesions are relatively scarce in experimental animals. In this context, these studies have been performed using acute resections or successive partial surgical ablations within a cerebral structure. For instance, in rats, it has been shown that major deficits are present 36 days after an acute ablation of the somatosensory cortex. These deficits were absent when the same area was removed in two stages [1]. In another study performed in cats, the animals fell into a deep coma and died within a few days after the acute resection of the midbrain reticular formation, in contrast with these animals that were injured gradually by means of several surgeries (up to eight) in which complete recovery was found [2]. The same pattern has been observed in monkeys, since acute ablations of the prefrontal cortex induce functional deficits that were more severe than these observed after serial lesions [3]. Furthermore, it has been discussed that the same type of dissociation is observed in humans, from data obtained from stroke and slow tumoural invasions [4].

Thus, it appears that the brain damage's sequelae are smaller in slow-growing than in acute lesions. It is important to take into account the type of lesion that the patient suffers in order to prescribe the adequate treatment. In this context, the recovery mechanism could differ between traumatic, stroke, or hypoxic-induced lesions.

However, it has been suggested that cortical damage induces motor deficits mediated by the inhibition of remote sites related into the injured region [5]. This inhibition could be maintained by the severity of the injury; then it would be expected that certain slow-growing lesions could maintain such inhibition for a much greater length of time than an acute lesion, in contrast with data described above.

The role of norepinephrine (NE) in recovery after brain injury has been widely documented [6, 7]. It has been reported that NE infusions into the cerebellum [8], and the administration of NEergic agonist, such as amphetamine [9], prevent the motor deficit associated with the injury. This fact has been also observed after the systemic administration of L-threo-3,4-dihydroxyphenylserine (L-DOPS), a NE precursor [10]. Some studies performed with microdialysis have shown that extracellular NE in the cerebellum decreased after brain injury [11]. There is no available data about the role of the pons in the NE changes observed in the cerebellum after brain injury. It is known that the pons contains the locus coeruleus (LC), the main NE reservoir in the central nervous system [12]. There are anatomical relationships between the LC, the motor cortex and the cerebellum [13, 14]). Regarding these facts, we described an increase of NE in the pons after 6 hours following the cortical ablation [15] that could be related to the motor impairment measured by the footprint analysis. This could be an example of an acute injury in experimental animals. In this work, we evaluate the effects of the Fe2Cl-induced lesion in the motor cortex, as an example of slow-growing lesion, the pontine and cerebellar NE content, and then compared them with our results obtained using an ablation-induced injury, in order to clarify the mechanisms involved in the sequelae expression.

Materials and Methods

Sixty-five male wistar rats (280–320 g) provided by the vivarium of Instituto Nacional de Rehabilitacion were used. Animals were fed with Purina rodent laboratory chow and maintained on a 12–12 light–darkness schedule. Rats were adapted to the laboratory conditions at least 1 week prior to the surgeries. During this time, rats were handled daily in order to habituate them to the experimental manipulations, and a training protocol was performed that entailed waling along a wooden walkway covered with a paper strip (6.8 cm wide X 100 cm length) in order to obtain traces of their footprints (Figure 1), as described by Gonzalez-Pina et al. [15]. Rats were treated according to the *Guide for the Care and Use of Experimental Animals* [16]. We used the minimal possible number of animals using bioethical and statistical criteria, according to Festing [17].

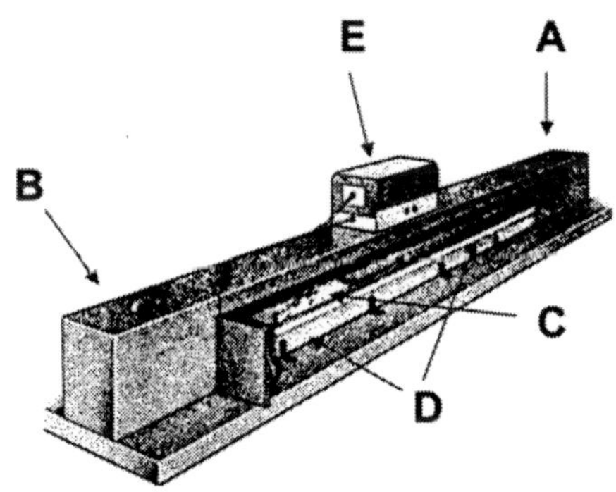

Figure 1. Scheme of the walkway used to perform the motor evaluations. A. Starting cage. B. Finishing cage. C. Rat walking through the walkway on a paper strip placed on the walkway floor. The rats had their extremities stained in order to record their footprints. D. Metallic plates where mild electrical shocks were administrated during the training phase of the study. E. Electroshock device. (Courtesy of D.I. Gonzalo Gonzalez-Pina).

Rats were allocated into six groups: sham-operated A (SA; n=11), sham-operated B (SB), injured by cortical ablation (CA), injured by cortical ablation and recovering (CAR), injured by Fe2Cl intraparenchimal injection in the motor cortex (Fe), and injured by the same procedure and recovering (FeR).

Twenty-four hours after the surgeries, a basal record of the footprint was taken in all the rats. In order to perform the surgeries, animals were anesthetized with Ketamine–Xylazine (100 mg/kg–5 mg/kg). Then, the rats were mounted in a stereotaxic frame (David Kopf). The skull was exposed by means of an incision on the scalp and a trephine hole was performed (1 mm diameter, approximately) upon the cortical site representative of the hindlimb [18], located in the following coordinates: posterior 2 mm and lateral 2 mm with respect to the bregma. Some of the rats were injured in the right hindlimb motor area (MCx) by means of the aspiration of such tissue using a vacuum pump (Stoelting 6C) coupled to a glass pipette (1 mm diameter), in the CA (N=6) and CAR (n=12) groups, while all the procedures without aspiration were performed in the SA (n=11) group. Then, once animals recovered from the anesthetic effects, the footprints were recorded every 6 hours for 48 hours. In the remaining subjects, a cannula directed to the MCx was surgically placed in the SB (n=16), Fe (n=5) and FeR (n=16) groups and fixed with dental acrylic. Once these animals were recovering from surgery, artificial cerebrospinal fluid (CSF, 5μl) was injected in free-moving conditions in the SB animals, while CSF containing Fe2Cl (50 mM) was injected to the Fe and FeR groups. Then, the footprint recording was performed each 24 hours for 20 days. The rats of the Fe group were sacrificed by decapitation 2 days after the intraparenchimal Fe2Cl injection was administrated.

At the end of the recording periods, the remaining groups of rats were sacrificed by decapitation and the left and right sides of the pons and cerebella were removed. The full brain was placed on a cool plate in order to extract the pons and cerebellum, each divided into right and left sides. Tissues were collected in teflon tubes and a solution of 0.5 ml of perchloric acid 0.4 N containing 0.1% w/v of sodium metabisulfite was added. Then the tissues were homogenized and centrifuged at 15,000 rpm for 10 minutes at 4°C. The supernatant was filtered and stored at –70°C for chromatographic analysis. The content of NE was analyzed by high performance liquid chromatography (HPLC, Perkin-Elmer LC-250) coupled to a metrohom electrochemical detector. The peaks were sent to a computer with a Perkin-Elmer 1020 Plus program. In order to determine the concentrations of NE, the chromatograms of the samples were interpolated with the chromatogram obtained from four standard samples, whose NE concentrations were known. An analytical column for catecholamines was used (ALLTECH, adsorbosphere C18 100 X 4.8 mm, 3 μm of particle size). The mobile phase utilized consisted of a phosphate buffer solution (0.1 mM, pH 3.2) that contained (in mM): sodium octyl sulfate (0.2), EDTA (0.1) and methanol (15% v/v). The flow rate employed was 1.2 ml/min while the potential was set at 0.65 V against a reference electrode of Ag/AgCl.

The encephalus was placed in a 10% formalin-buffer solution in order to delineate the lesion by means of the Kluver–Barrera stain. Following observation by light microscopy, the cavity was outlined on schemes taken from the Paxinos and Watson's stereotaxic atlas [19].

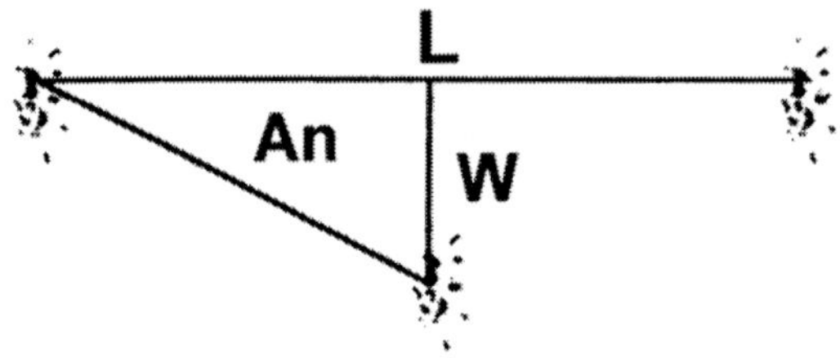

Figure 2. Stride's parameters measured in a typical footprint. L stride´s length (in cm), W=stride's width (in cm) and A=stride's angle (in grades).

Comparison between values obtained from the footprint analysis (length, width and anlge's stride, Figure 2) were performed using the Mann-Whitney U test (p=0.05), while an ANOVA was used in order to compare the means obtained from the total NE contents (p=0.05).

Results

After the cerebral coronal slices were processed, we observed that the cavity corresponding to the rats with ablation started –1.60 mm from the bregma (Figure 3A), increased to a maximum between –2.56 mm and –2.80 mm (Figure 3B), and then decreased to a final size between –3.14 mm and –3.60 mm (Figure 3C), covering the entire motor hindlimb cortical representation, according to Hall and Lindholm [18]. On the other hand, rats injured with Fe2Cl showed a track located inside the motor cortex approximately in 1.5 mm of depth, at –2 mm from bregma. These observations were performed in rats 2 days (Figure 4A) and 20 days (Figure 4B) post-injection.

Footprint analysis showed that all ablation-induced injury animals had a significant decrease in the stride's length after 6 hours (–8.00% ± 2.4; $P \leq 0.001$; Figure 5A), with a concomitant increase in the stride's angle (22.11% ± 4.65; $P \leq 0.003$; Figure 5B), while the stride's width did not show any significant change. As shown in these figures, recovery was observed 24 hours following injury, since the mean percentage of change with respect to the baseline was not significant when the SA group was compared with the CAR group. Such a recovery was sustained for 48 hours post-lesion. In contrast, the animals injured with Fe2Cl intraparenchimal administration (Figure 6) showed a significant increase in the stride´s length in days 2-3 following injection (12–18%; $P \leq 0.0086$) and a decrease in the stride's angle in days 2 (–5.24 ± 3.08; $P \leq 0.013$), 3 (–8% ± 3.13; $P \leq 0.021$), 4 (–5.5% ± 2.87; $P \leq 0.014$) and 5 (–3.3% ± 1.19; $P \leq 0.007$)

When the mean total content of NE was analyzed in either the right or left pontine sides, it was found that CA rats (6 hours following ablation-induced injury) showed a significant increase (in ng/g of fresh tissue) in NE (9.76 ± 0.72) in the right side when they were compared with SA (6.76 ± 0.87) and CAR (6.32 ± 0.71) groups. The same pattern of change was found in the left side ($P \leq 0.017$). There were no significant differences between NE levels found in both pontine sides in individual rats. Therefore, cerebellar NE content did not show any significant difference between the right ($P \leq 0.723$) and left ($P \leq 0.565$) hemispheres (Table 1).

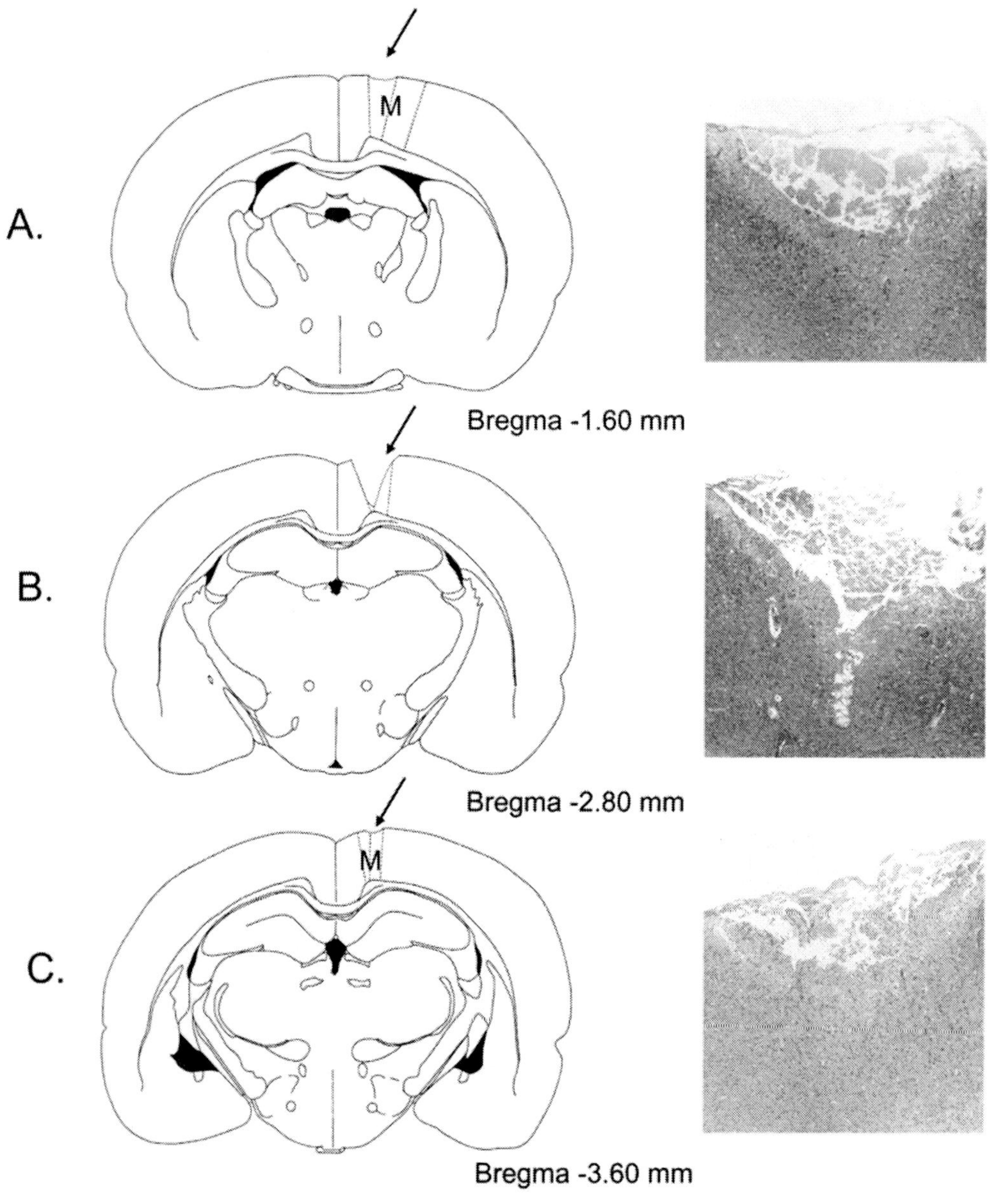

Figure 3. Schematic representation showing the extent of the lesions (left), and microphotographs (10x) taken from the equivalent places in one typical slice (right). After the microscopic observations were performed, the cavity was outlined on the equivalent schematics taken from the Paxinos and Watson's stereotaxic atlas [19]. It is observed in both schematics and photomicrographs that the lesion was circumscribed by the motor cortex in the hindlimb representative area. In A and C, the primary motor cortex border was affected (M), while in the injured area, a portion of the somatosensory cortex (B) was also affected. However, the lack of somatosensorial effects suggests that the size of the lesion in such an area was not significant (from Gonzalez-Pina et al. [21], with permission).

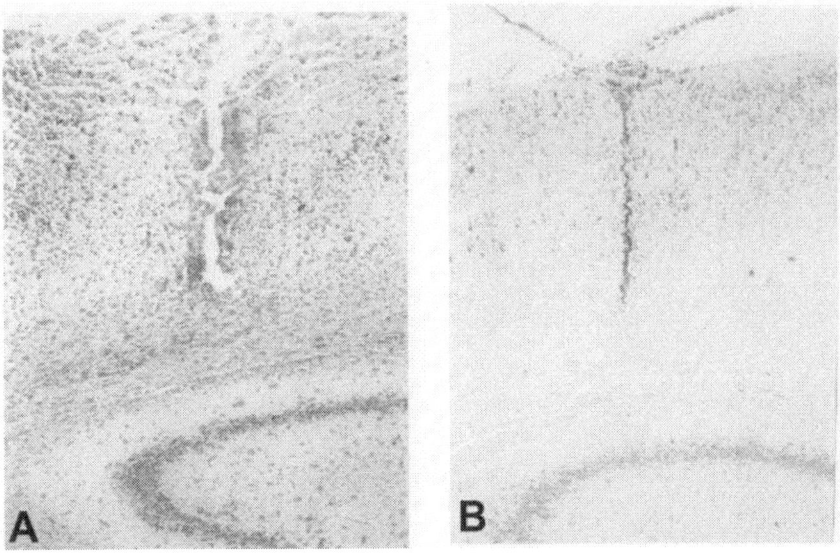

Figure 4. Representative slices showing the sites of intraparenchimal injection of Fe2Cl. The needle tip is shown at 1.5 mm of depth, in the hindlimb representative area of the motor cortex. (A) Two days following the injection. (B) Twenty days following the injection.

Table 1. Norepinephrine content (in ng/g of fresh tissue) found in pons and cerebellum, in sham-operated, injured by cortical ablation and recovering rats

PONS			
	Sham	Post-injury (6 h)	Post-injury (48 h)
Right side	7.17 ± 1.08	9.76 ± 0.72[a,b]	6.76 ± 0.87
Left side	7.30 ± 0.79	10.16 ± 0.78[a,b]	7.11 ± 0.99
CEREBELLUM			
Right hemisphere	7.26 ± 0.89	7.47 ± 0.77	7.40 ± 0.93
Left hemisphere	6.95 ± 1.03	8.46 ± 0.66	8.72 ± 1.25

[a] Significant with respect to sham

[b] Significant with respect to post-injury (48 hours)

Table 2. Norepinephrine content found (in ng/g of fresh tissue) in pons and cerebellum, in sham-operated, injured by Fe2Cl injection and in recovering rats

PONS			
	sham	Post-injury (2 days)	Post-injury (20 days)
Right side	3.12 ± 0.54	nd	2.75 ± 0.44
Left side	3.35 ± 0.97	nd	3.23 ± 0.58
CEREBELLUM			
Right hemisphere	7.11 ± 0.90	0.29 ± 0.18[a,b]	3.78 ± 1.88
Left hemisphere	7.10 ± 0.81	0.31 ± 0.19[a,b]	11.06 ± 4.87

nd=non-detectable amount.

[a] Significant with respect to sham.

[b] Significant with respect to post-injury (20 days).

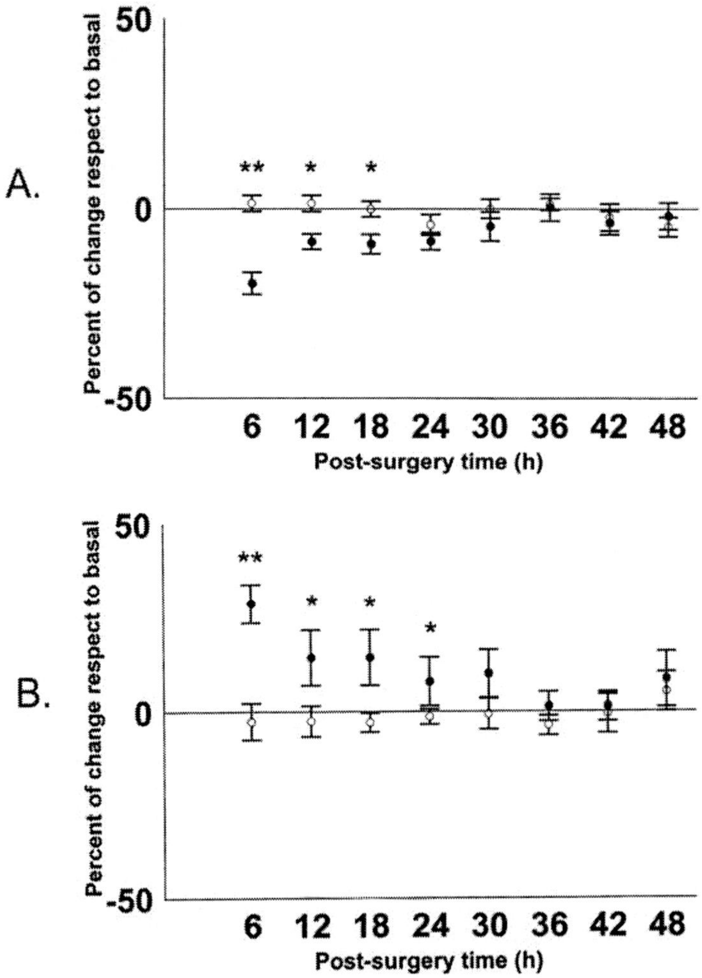

Figure 5. Parameters measured in the footprints. Since the stride's width did not show any significant differences, such data are not presented. (A) Percent of change with respect to baseline in the stride's length, measured every 6 hours for 48 hours post-surgery. An important decrease after 6 hours in injured animals was observed. Recovery was observed 24 hours post-lesion and was maintained over the next 24 hours. Data are expressed as mean ± s.e.m. Mann–Whitney's U (*$P \leq 0.05$, **$P \leq 0.01$). ○ Sham operated rats; ● injured rats. (B) Percent of change with respect to baseline in the stride's angle, where a significant increase after 6 hours post-lesion was observed. Recovery was observed 30 hours post-lesion, although after 24 hours a marginally significant difference was observed. Recovery was sustained for at least 48 hours. Results are expressed as mean ± s.e.m. Mann– Whitney's U (*$P \leq 0.05$, **$P \leq 0.01$). ○ Sham operated rats; ● injured rats (From Gonzalez-Pina et al. [21], with permission).

In the case of Fe2Cl-induced injury, it was found that the NE levels after 2 post-injury days are fully depleted in both, the right and left sides of the pons in the Fe group. However, in the FeR rats, the NE levels found in the right and the left sides were very similar to those observed in the SB rats. On the other hand, cerebellar NE content was found significantly decreased in both right ($p \leq 0.001$) and left ($p \leq 0.003$) hemispheres in the Fe rats, 2 days after the lesion was performed (Table 2).

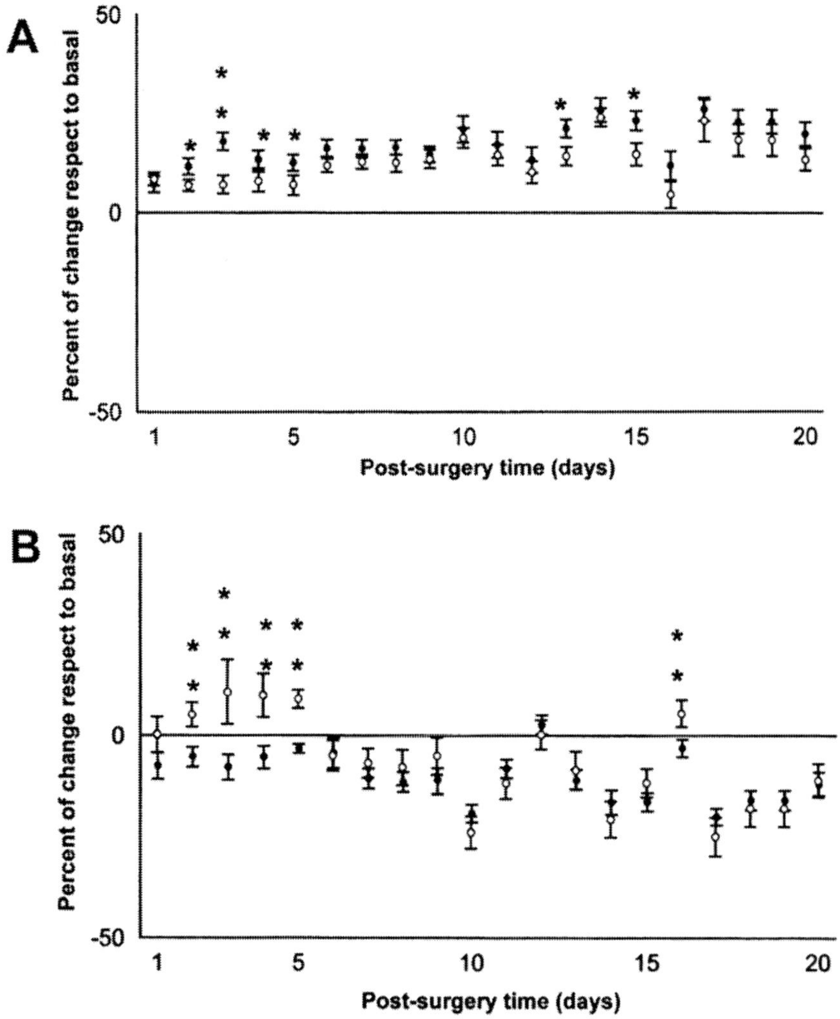

Figure 6. Parameters measured in the footprints. Since the stride's width did not show any significant differences, such data are not presented. (A) Percent of change with respect to baseline in the stride's length, measured every 24 h for 20 h post-lesion. An important increase after 2 h in injured animals was observed. Recovery was observed 6 days post-lesion and was maintained over the next 15 days, although some late sequels in days 13 and 15 were observed. Data are expressed as mean ± s.e.m. Mann– Whitney's U (*$P \leq 0.05$, **$P \leq 0.01$). ○ Sham operated rats; ● injured rats. (B) Percent of change with respect to baseline in the stride's angle, where a significant decrease after 2 days post-lesion was observed. Recovery was observed at day 6 post-lesion, although at day 16 a late sequel was observed. Results are expressed as mean ± s.e.m. Mann–Whitney's U (*$P \leq 0.05$, **$P \leq 0.01$). ○ Sham operated rats; ● injured rats.

Discussion

Footprint analysis and motor assessment showed that the variances in cerebral lesions induced differential effects on the pontine and cerebellar NE and on the stride's parameters. In the case of cortical ablation, NE content was elevated 6 hours after surgery, and when animals recovered, pontine NE content was found to have returned to levels similar to those found in sham-operated rats after 48 hours of surgery. On the other hand, NE was fully depleted in the pons 2 days after the animals were injured by Fe2Cl, while after 20 days following injury it had returned to normal levels. This fact was observed in both sides of the pons. It is known that innervation from the LC to the MCx is ipsilateral [14]. Thus, it is to be expected that an injury in the MCx will produce an ipsilateral effect on the LC. However, we found the changes in NE in both sides of the pons. There is strong evidence that behavioral effects of motor cortical injury results from functional depression in remote but intact brain areas related to the injured site, a concept known as diaschisis [20]. This seems to be applicable in the case of a slow-growing lesion, where NE decreases when the motor impairment is higher. In the case of acute lesion (cortical ablation), NE increase in the pons could be also part of such functional depression, as we have previously proposed [21], as a norepinephrinergic pontine autoinhibitory mechanism.

Our results suggest that diaschisis is involved, despite the mechanisms implied, because we have the presence of a cerebral injury circumscribed, a neuronal basis for the functional depression, the participation of a remote structure related with the lesion site (the pons), anatomical relationships between the pons and the cortex, and the process is reversible [30].

In this context, pharmacological studies suggest that inhibition of NE release on postsynaptic target cells could be mediated by the α2-adrenoceptors [22,23], widely distributed in the LC neurons. Thus, the binding of pontine NE to such receptors in the LC, enhanced by the observed NE increase, could produce the decreased NE release previously reported in cerebellum after MCx injury, as assessed by microdialysis [11]. Specifically, the α2A-receptor subtype could be involved, since it is found in 100% of the rat's LC neurons [24]; and, it has been reported that an α2-receptor agonist inhibited release of NE by 96% [25]. The inhibitory action of NE has also been observed in other brain areas, such as the acetylcholine NE-induced inhibition in the tegmental nuclei [26].

Thus, we face two mechanisms of diaschisis. One could be mediated by depletion in pontine NE, perhaps as a consequence of the reconstruction of the damaged circuits produced by the oxidative stress brought on by the Fe2Cl administration. It is possible that the NEergic neurons must synthesize proteins instead of NE, in order to rebuild the damaged axons. On the other hand, acute injury produces a NE increase that also could lead to inhibition, this time mediated by the α-receptors. Both mechanisms cause motor impairments that are consistent with the motor assessment. Footprint analysis showed that the stride's length decreased in CA animals while it increased in Fe animals, when NE levels increased and decreased, respectively. It was also observed that stride´s angle increased in CA animals while it decreased in Fe rats. Thus, a negative relationship between NE content in the pons and stride's length, and a positive relationship between NE content and stride´s angle is apparent.

It is unclear how unilateral cortical injury results in bilateral increase of total NE levels in the pons, since innervation between the LC and cortex is predominantly ipsilateral [14]. It is possible that the effects of the unilateral MCx injury have an influence on both pontine sides [11]. Instead, the LC innervation of the cerebellum is bilateral [27], and the effects of MCx injury in the cerebellum may lead to bilateral retrograde effects within the LC neurons. However, we have not observed changes in the cerebellar NE levels. Most of the literature has shown that cerebellar NE is involved in the mechanisms leading to recovery. A decrease in cerebellar NE has been reported after cortical injury [8, 11], and such levels return to normal values when amphetamine is administered [6, 8]. It has also been reported that cerebellar NE infusions facilitate recovery after sensorimotor cortex injury [8]. Such facts strongly support a cerebellum NE-mediated mechanism to achieve recovery after brain injury. The absence of changes in cerebellar NE content found in rats injured by ablation indicates that NE activity in the cerebellum related to recovery from motor cortical ablation is confined to discrete regions, such as the cerebellar cortex. It is known that the ventral and dorsal portions of the LC innervate all of the neurons of the cerebellar cortex and, to a lesser extent, the cerebellar nuclei [28, 29]. However, the extent of the damage could be amplified in the case of a slow-growing lesion, because the Fe injured rats showed an important increase of NE after 2 post-lesion days.

Thus, we demonstrate that motor impairment depends of the kind of injury, and that remote functional inhibition could be mediated by differential effects on pontine NE. On the other hand, we found that when motor performance is recovered, animals showed pontine NE levels very similar to these found in sham-operated rats 48 hours following surgery, suggesting an important role of the pons in the cerebellar inhibition after cortical injury, previously reported by others. Therefore, lack of effects on cerebellar NE content after ablation opens the need to search for specific cerebellar areas related to recovery after cortical brain injury. This also applies to the global cerebellar decrease observed after Fe2Cl-induced injury, since a generalized depletion of NE could lead to a major behavioral disfunction, such as ataxic symptoms and balance impairments.

The relevance of this study of the biochemical mechanisms leading to recovery after brain injury is pertinent to the development of pharmacological strategies that enhance recovery in humans. It must be noted that the results of clinical experience are very similar to those observed in experimental animals [31], suggesting that the mechanisms observed in the basic research are comparable between rats and humans.

Finally, it must be regarded that the clinical use of NE agonists and antagonists, such as antidepressants and ansiolytics in humans after stroke, could alleviate or extend to remote neuronal depression, facilitating or hindering functional recovery. More studies are needed in order to elucidate the detailed mechanisms underlying brain recovery after injury. In particular, the specific role of LC in the norepinephrinergic functional depression must be clarified.

References

[1] Finger S, Marshak RA, Cohen M, Scheff S, Trace R, Niemand D. (1971) Effects of successive and simultaneous lesions of somatosensory cortex on tactile discrimination in the rat. *J Comp Physiol Psychol, 77*, 221-7.

[2] Adametz J. (1959). Rate of recovery of functioning in cats with rostral reticular lesions; an experimental study. *J Neurosurg, 16*, 85-97.

[3] Rosen J, Stein D, Butters N. (1971). Recovery of function after serial ablation of prefrontal cortex in the rhesus monkey. *Science, 173*, 353-6.

[4] Desmurget M, Bonnetblanc FC, and Duffau H. (2007). Contrasting acute and slow-growing lesions: a new door to brain plasticity *Brain. 130*, 898-914.

[5] Nudo RJ, Plautz EJ, Frost SB. (2001). Role of adaptive plasticity in recovery of function after damage to motor cortex. *Muscle &Nerve, 24*, 8: 1000-1019.

[6] Goldstein LB. (1989) Amphetamine-facilitated functional recovery after stroke. In: Ginsberg MD, Dietrich WD, eds. *Cerebrovascular Diseases: Sixteenth Research (Princeton) Conference*. New York, NY: Raven Press, 303–308.

[7] Godstein LB. (2003). Neuropharmacology of TBI- induced plasticity. *Brain Injury, 17*, 685-694.

[8] Boyeson MG, Krobert KA. (1992). Cerebellar norepinephrine infusions facilitate recovery after sensorimotor cortex injury. *Brain Res Bull, 29*, 435-439.

[9] Sutton RL, Hovda DA, Chen MJ, Feeney DM. (2000). Alleviation of brain injury-induced cerebral metabolic depression by amphetamine: a cytochrome oxidase histochemistry study. *Neural Plast, 7*, 109-125.

[10] Kikuchi K, Nishino K Ohyu H. (2000). Increasing CNS norepinephrine levels by the precursor L-DOPS facilitates beam-walking recovery after sensorimotor cortex ablation in rats. *Brain Res, 860*, 130-135.

[11] Krobert KA, Sutton RL , Feeney DM. (1994). Spontaneous and amphetamine-evoked release of cerebellar noradrenaline after sensorimotor cortex contusion: an in vivo microdialysis study in the awake rat. *J. Neurochem 62*, 2233-2240.

[12] Berridge, CW. and Waterhouse, BD. (2003). The locus coeruleus-noradrenergic system: modulation of behavioral state and state-dependent cognitive processes. *Review. Brain Res, 42*, 33-84.

[13] Cicirata F. Zappalà A. Serapide MF. Parenti R. Pantò MR, Paz C. (2005). Different pontine projections to the two sides of the cerebellum. Review. *Brain Res, 49*, 280-294.

[14] Steindler DA, (1981). Locus coeruleus neurons have axons that branch to the forebrain and cerebellum. (1981). *Brain Res, 223*, 367-373.

[15] Gonzalez-Pina R. Bueno-Nava A. Montes S, Alfaro-Rodriguez A, Gonzalez-Maciel A. Reynoso-Robles and Ayala-Guerrero F. (2005). Pontine norepinephrine content alter motor cortical ablation in rats. *Proc. West. Pharmacol. Soc. 48*, 73-76.

[16] Olfert ED, Cross BM, McWilliam AA. (1993). Guide for the care and use of experimental animals. *Can Council Animal Care, 1*, 211.

[17] Festing MFW. (1994). Reduction of animal use: experimental design and quality of experiments. *Lab Anim Sci, 28*, 212-221.

[18] Hall RD, Lindholm EP. (1974). Organization of motor and somatosensory neocortex in albino-rat. *Brain Research, 66*, 23.

[19] Paxinos G, Watson C. (1982). The rat brain in stereotaxi coordinates. *Academi Press, Australia.*

[20] Serteser M, Ösben T, Gümüslü S, Balkan S, Balkan E. (2001). Biochemical evidence of crossed cerebellar diaschisis in terms of nitric oxide indicators and lipid peroxidation products in rats durin gocal cerebral ischemia. *Acta neurol Scand, 103*, 43-48.

[21] Gonzalez-Pina R, Bueno-Nava A, Montes S, Alfaro-Rodriguez A, Gonzalez-Maciel A, Reynoso-Robles R, Ayala-Guerrero F. (2006). Pontine and Cerebellar Norepinephrine Content in Adult Rats Recoverin from Focal Cortical Injury. *Neurochem Res, 31,* 443-1449.

[22] Washburn M, Moises HC. (1989). Electrophysiological correlates of presynaptic alpha 2-receptor mediated inhibition of norepinephrine relase at locus coeruleus synapses in dentate gyrus. *J Neuroscide, 9*, 2131-2140.

[23] Nasseri A, Minneman KP. (1987). Relationship between alpha 2-adrenergic receptor bindin sites and the functional receptors inhibiting norepinephrine relase in rat cerebral cortex. *Mol Pharmacol, 32*, 655-662.

[24] Smeets WJ, Gonzalez A. (2000). Catecholamine system in the brain of vertebrates: new perspectives through a comparative approach. *Brain Res Rev, 33*, 308-379.

[25] Bucheller MM, Hadamek KK, Hein L. (2002). Two alpha (2)-adrenergic receptor subtypes, alpha(2A and alpha (2C), inhibit transmitter release in the brain of gene targeted mice. *Neuroscience, 109*, 819-826.

[26] Hobson JA, McCarley RW. (1977) The brain as a dream state generator: an activation synthesis hypothesis of the dream process. *Am J Psychiatry, 134*, 1335-1348.

[27] Room P, Postema F, Korf J. (1981) Divergent axon collaterals of rat locus coeruleus neurons: demonstration by a fluorescent double labeling technique. *Brain Res, 221*, 219-230.

[28] Schambra UB, Mackensen GB, Stafford.Smith M, Haines DE, Schwinn DA. (2005) Neuron specific alfa-adrenergic receptor expression in human cerebellum: implication for emerging cerebellar roles in neurologic disease. *Neuroscience, 135*, 507-523.

[29] Schweighofer N, Doya K, Kuroda S, (2004). Cerebelar aminergic neuromodulation: towards a functional understanding. *Brain Res Rev, 44*, 103-116.

[30] Feeney DM, Baron JC. Diaschisis. (1986). *Stroke 17*, 817-830

[31] Godstein LB. (2000). Effects of amphetamines and small related molecules on recovery after stroke in animals and man. Neuropharmacology, *39*, 852-859.

In: Research Progress on Epinephrine ISBN: 978-1-60456-443-3
Editors: A. G. Lawson and R. I. Gorman, pp.129-146

Chapter VII

Differential Epinephrine and Norepinephrine Release from the Sympathectomized Rat Heart Compartments

Jitka Kuncová*[*], *Jitka Švíglerová*, *Šárka Faitová*, *Jan Capouch* and *Jana Slavíková
Department of Physiology, Medical School Plzeň, Charles University, Czech Republic

Abstract

Epinephrine in the heart is believed to be taken up mainly from the circulation by sympathetic nerve endings. However, at least three additional sources of epinephrine in the mammalian heart have been suggested to date: 1. Intrinsic ganglion neurons displaying phenylethanolamine N-methyltransferase (PNMT)-immunoreactivity, enzyme decisive in epinephrine synthesis; 2. Intrinsic cardiac adrenergic cells distinct from adrenergic neurons; 3. Myocardial cells containing inducible PNMT or nonspecific N-methyltransferase.

The aim of the study presented in this chapter was to evaluate epinephrine and norepinephrine release from the atria and left ventricles of rats subjected to neonatal chemical sympathectomy by guanethidine in comparison to age-matched controls.

At the age of 8 months, the heart atria or left ventricles were dissected, sliced, pooled and transferred into 12 parallelly perfused perfusion chambers. Tissues were superfused with oxygenated Krebs-Henseleit (KH) solution. After 40 min equilibration period, basal release of catecholamines was measured and then norepinephrine or epinephrine outflows were stimulated by depolarization with 50 mmol/l KCl in the superfusion fluid. Norepinephrine and epinephrine concentrations in superfusates were determined using radioimmunoassay ultrasensitive diagnostic kits. The effects of

[*] E-mail: jitka.kuncova@lfp.cuni.cz

tyramine (10^{-6} mol/l), desipramine (10^{-7} mol/l), and dibutyryl cAMP (10^{-4} mol/l) were tested in the atria and left ventricles. In addition, resting heart rate and blood pressure were measured bimonthly and epinephrine and norepinephrine concentrations were determined in the heart compartments of control and guanethidine-treated animals at the ages of 4 and 8 months.

At the age of 8 months, the tissue concentrations of norepinephrine in the denervated atria and left ventricles did not exceed 20% and 10% of the control values, respectively. In contrast, epinephrine concentrations did not significantly differ between guanethidine- and vehicle-treated preparations.

Basal release of norepinephrine from the control samples was significantly enhanced by depolarization (high KCl), dibutyryl cAMP, tyramine and desipramine. Stimulated norepinephrine release (high KCl) was significantly higher in the presence of tyramine, desipramine and dibutyryl cAMP. Basal release of norepinephrine from the sympathectomized heart was significantly lower than that from the control preparations and it was enhanced by tyramine, desipramine and cAMP. In contrast, epinephrine release from the denervated atria and ventricles was not affected by depolarization, tyramine and desipramine, but it was significantly increased by dibutyryl cAMP.

Our results provide further evidence of epinephrine signaling system independent of the sympathetic innervation in the mammalian heart. Epinephrine release from non-neuronal sources might help to maintain cardiac functions in the absence of sympathetic innervation.

Introduction

Epinephrine [adrenaline; 3,4-Dihydroxy-α-(methylaminomethyl)benzyl alcohol] is a monoamine derived from the amino acid tyrosine that is converted by tyrosine hydroxylase (TH) to dihydroxyphenylalanine (DOPA). Decarboxylation of DOPA by aromatic amino acid decarboxylase (AADC) gives rise dopamine that is hydroxylated to norepinephrine by dopamine β-hydoxylase (DβH). Epinephrine is synthesized via methylation of the primary distal amine of norepinephrine by phenylethanolamine N-methyltransferase (PNMT).

Epinephrine is a major catecholamine secreted from the adrenal medulla in response to various physiological and pathological stimuli such as mental stress, threatening, exciting, or environmental stressor conditions [1]. It contributes by more than 90% to circulating epinephrine [2]. However, small amounts of epinephrine are present in most peripheral tissues [3-5]. The intracardiac epinephrine was believed to be taken up from the circulation into the sympathetic nerve endings via norepinephrine transporter [6].

However, recent experimental evidence suggests that both catecholamines are distributed in the mammalian heart in at least three additional sources: 1. Intrinsic ganglion neurons of the cardiac nerve plexus that are capable of operating with some degree of independence from extrinsic neuronal inputs [7, 8] express TH, DβH and PNMT, i.e. the enzymatic machinery necessary for norepinephrine and epinephrine synthesis [9]. In the rat heart, the cell bodies of ganglion neurons are located in the atria, particularly the left one, but not in the ventricles [10, 11]. 2. Intrinsic catecholaminergic (ICA) cells that are diffusely distributed throughout the heart including both atria and ventricles contribute to the total cardiac content of norepinephrine and epinephrine by 18%, and 13%, respectively [12]. ICA cells do not have neuronal or chromaffin cell ultrastructural morphology on electron microscopic analysis and are capable of catecholamine uptake and release [13]. 3. There is also compelling evidence that myocardial cells contain PNMT mRNA that can be regulated by stress in a glucocorticoid-dependent manner [14, 15]. Negligible portion of norepinephrine in the atria could be localized in two additional cell types: small intensely fluorescent (SIF) cells and glomus-like bodies (GLB) displaying moderate or week DβH immunoreactivity, respectively, suggesting the presence of norepinephrine [16].

Guanethidine is a neurotoxin widely used to induce permanent sympathectomy in newborn and adult rats [17]. It was clinically used as an antihypertensive drug since it is a substrate of norepinephrine transporter; it is taken up into the sympathetic terminals where it replaces norepinephrine thus interfering with its release and effects. The mechanism of guanethidine induced sympathectomy involves an autoimmune response. Ultrastructural morphological events include a gross swelling of the mitochondria followed by lymphocyte infiltration and subsequent degeneration of neuronal cell mediated most probably by the natural killer cells.

Although adrenal medullary cells express norepinephrine transporter, they are not susceptible to the toxic effect of guanethidine [18]. The expression of the norepinephrine transporter in the ICA cells was also documented [13]; however, their sensitivity to the sympatholytic drugs has not been studied yet.

The aim of the present study was to evaluate epinephrine and norepinephrine release from the atria and left ventricles of rats subjected to neonatal chemical sympathectomy by guanethidine. After neonatal sympathectomy, the blood pressure, resting heart rate and the effect of β-adrenergic antagonist on the heart rate were measured at the ages of 2, 4, 6, and 8 months to verify the effectivity of the chemical sympathectomy. At the age of 8 months, the heart atria or left ventricles were dissected, sliced and norepinephrine and epinephrine outflows were studied under basal conditions and after depolarization of tissues by high potassium ion concentration in the superfusion solution. The effects of a substrate of norepinephrine transporter tyramine, norepinephrine transporter inhibitor desipramine and dibutyryl cAMP were tested.

Our results provide further evidence of non-sympathetic norepinephrine and epinephrine pools in the mammalian heart. Catecholamine release from extraneuronal sources might help to regulate cardiac performance in pathological situations associated with deteriorated function of the sympathetic innervation.

Methods

All experiments were conducted in accordance with European Directive for the Protection of Vertebrate Animals Used for Experimental and Other Scientific Purposes (86/609/EU), the relevant Guidelines of the Czech Ministry of Agriculture for scientific experimentation on animals and were approved by the University Committee for Experiments on Laboratory Animals (Charles University, Czech Republic).

Animals

Pregnant Wistar rats purchased from VELAZ (Prague, Czech Republic) were housed individually with free access to food and water. On the day of birth (designated as postnatal day 0), pups were randomly divided into two groups: The guanethidine-treated rats received subcutaneously guanethidine sulfate (50 mg/kg) dissolved in 0.9% NaCl solution on postnatal days 1-21. The control animals were injected with equal volumes of solvent at the same time points. Before weaning (four weeks after birth), 7-9 pups were kept with one nursing dam and then the animals were housed five *per* cage, fed standard laboratory chow *ad libitum* with free access to drinking water. All male rats were used for further experiments at the ages of 4 and 8 months.

Measurement of Systolic and Diastolic Blood Pressures

Blood pressure (systolic and diastolic) was measured at the age of two months and then bimonthly by a non-invasive tail-cuff method using an RTBP apparatus (Kent Scientific Co., CT, USA). The rat was placed into a restrainer and its tail was inserted into the occlusion and plethysmographic cuffs. The pressure was first raised to 200 mmHg and then slowly released. Blood pressure values were derived from an average of 10-15 measurements per animal at each time point. Two preliminary training sessions were performed during 2 weeks before final blood pressure determinations.

Measurement of the Heart Rate

To estimate the tonic influence of the cardiac sympathetic innervation on the heart rate, the animals were placed in a small chamber with electrodes in the floor that were connected to electrocardiograph (EKG Seiva Praktik, Prague, Czech Republic). Animals were let to adapt for 20 min and then the resting heart rate was measured four times in one-minute intervals. Non-specific β-adrenergic receptor antagonist metipranolol (Hoechst-Biotika, Martin, Slovac Republic; 2 mg/kg of body weight) was injected subcutaneously after previous administration of muscarinic receptor antagonist atropine (atropine sulfate, Sigma Aldrich, Prague, Czech Republic; 4 mg/kg, s.c.) and the heart rate was measured again. The values mentioned in the results represent means of these measurements.

Measurement of Norepinephrine and Epinephrine Release in Vitro

Rats were anaesthetized with ether and decapitated. The hearts were rapidly removed and placed into ice-cold oxygenated Krebs-Henseleit (KH) solution of the following composition (in mmol/l): NaCl 113, $NaHCO_3$ 25, KCl 4.75, $CaCl_2$ 2.5, $MgSO_4$ 1.19, glucose 11.1, Na_2EDTA 0.029, and ascorbic acid 0.289. Both atria or the left ventricles were dissected, sliced, pooled (approx. 40-60 mg of atrial tissue and 100-200 mg of left ventricular tissue) and transferred into 0.5 ml perfusion chambers. Tissues were superfused at a rate of 0.1 ml/min with oxygenated (95% O_2/5% CO_2) KH solution. All perfusion experiments were performed at 37°C according to the scheme shown in Figure 1A. Norepinephrine release from the control atria in the preliminary experiment is shown in Figure 1B. After a 40 min equilibration period, seven 10 min fractions were collected at 0°C. Spontaneous release of norepinephrine was measured in fractions 1 and 5 (B1 and B2 respectively), i.e. in the course of perfusion by the KH solution containing 4.75 mmol/l KCl. After collection of B1 and B2 fractions, catecholamine outflow was stimulated by depolarization with a superfusion fluid containing 50 mmol/l KCl, in which the concentration of NaCl was reduced by 50 mmol/l, and catecholamine concentrations were measured in fractions 3 and 7 (S1 and S2 respectively), i.e. in the course of perfusion by the modified KH solution containing 50 mmol/l KCl.

The effect of the neuronal uptake blocker desipramine (Sigma Aldrich, Prague, Czech Republic) on norepinephrine outflow was tested using a similar experimental protocol in both groups of animals at concentration 10^{-7} mol/l. Spontaneous and stimulated norepinephrine outputs were measured in the absence (fractions B1 and S1) and presence of desipramine (fractions $B2_{DES}$ and $S2_{DES}$) in the superfusion fluid.

Similarly, the effects of tyramine and dibutyryl cAMP (Sigma Aldrich, Prague, Czech Republic) on the basal and KCl-stimulated catecholamine outflows were studied using the same experimental protocol. Norepinephrine and epinephrine concentrations in the superfusates were determined using ultrasensitive radioimmunoassay diagnostic kits (LDN, Hamburg, FRG).

Extraction of Catecholamines

Control and guanethidine-treated rats at the ages of 4 and 8 months were anaesthetized with ether and killed by decapitation. The hearts were rapidly excised, rinsed with ice-cold saline and freed of connective tissue and fat. Right and left atria and free walls of both ventricles were dissected and immediately frozen on dry ice and weighed.

Norepinephrine and epinephrine were extracted from the heart compartments by homogenization in 10 volumes of 0.1 mol/l HCl containing 1% of ascorbic acid and subsequent centrifugation (10,000 *g*, 4°C, 20 min). Supernatants were diluted 1:10 with distilled water and stored at -75°C until RIA. Norepinephrine and epinephrine concentrations were assayed in tissue extracts by RIA using commercial kits (IBL Hamburg, FRG).

Data Analysis

Results are presented as mean ± SEM. Statistical differences were tested by unpaired two-tailed Student's t-test or by analysis of variance (ANOVA) followed by post hoc Fisher's Least Significant Difference test, using software package STATISTICA Cz, version 7 (StatSoft CR, Prague, Czech Republic). Normality of populations and homogeneity of variances were tested before each ANOVA. The results were considered significantly different when $p < 0.05$.

A

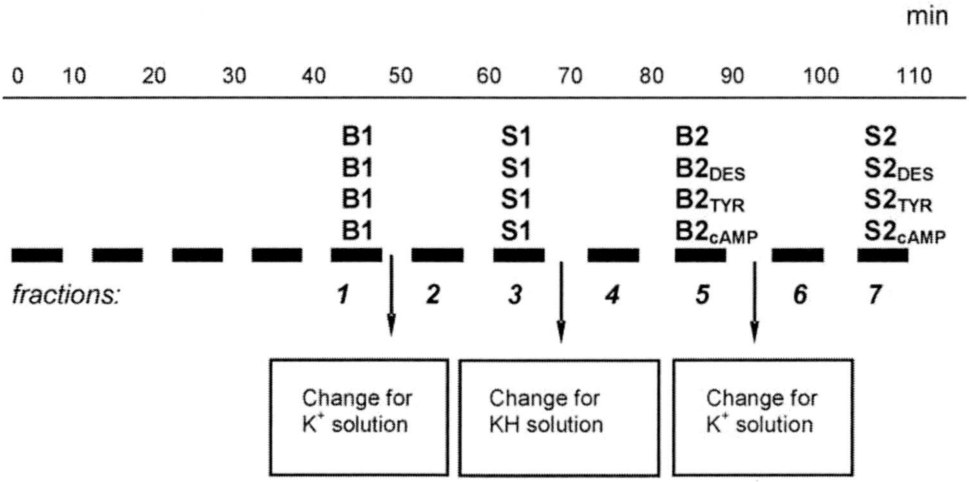

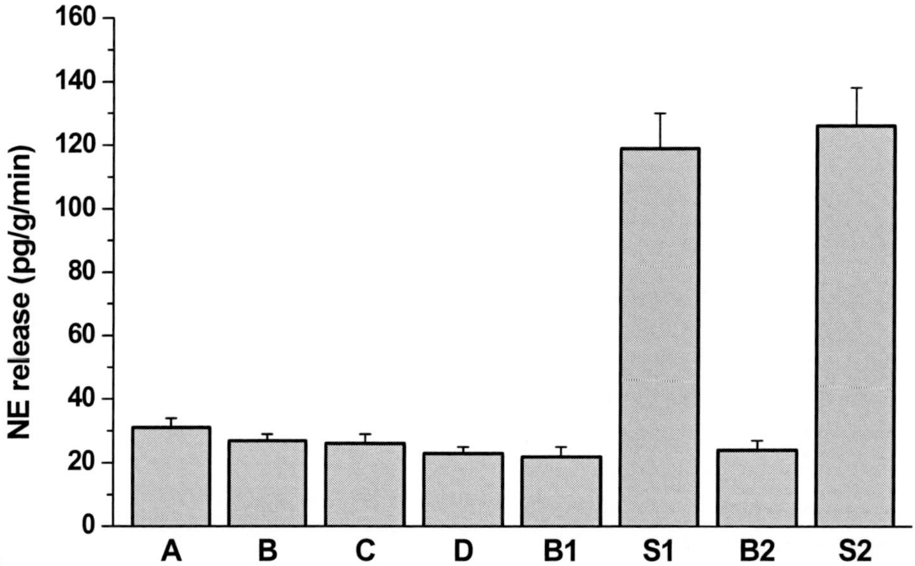

B

Figure 1A: The scheme of the superfusion protocol. Perfusion chambers contained sliced atria of 8-month-old rats (40 – 60 mg tissue per chamber). After a 40-min equilibration period, 10-min fractions were collected. Immediately after the collection of fractions B1 and B2 (fraction No 1 and 5), in which spontaneous norepinephrine outflow was measured, the superfusion fluid was changed for a solution containing 50 mmol/l KCl, and after 10-min mixed outflow (fraction No 2 and 6), another 10-min stimulated fractions (S1 and S2) were collected (fraction No 3 and 7). The indices describe substances present in the superfusion media: DES = desipramine (10^{-7} mol/l), TYR = tyramine (10^{-6} mol/l), cAMP = dibutyryl cyclic AMP (10^{-4} mol/l).

B: Norepinephrine release from the heart atria in the control experiment expressed in pg/g/min (n = 6). The four 10-min intervals during the equilibration period are designated A, B, C, and D.

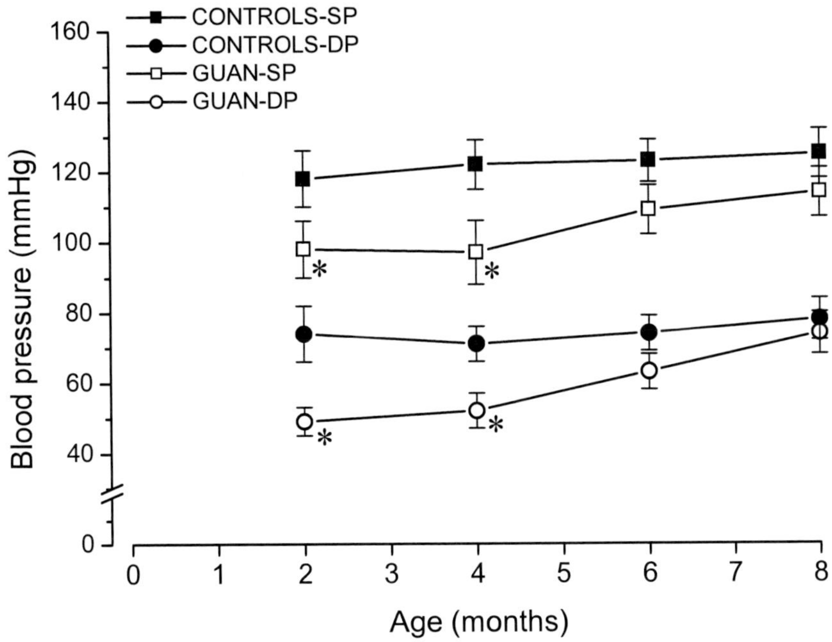

Figure 2. Systolic (SP) and diastolic blood pressures (BP) in control (CONTROLS; closed symbols; n = 8) and sympathectomized rats (GUAN; open symbols; n = 8) at the ages of 2, 4, 6, and 8 months. Data are displayed as mean ± SEM. *$p < 0.05$, compared to the respective control value.

Results

Blood Pressure

As shown in figure 2, sympathectomized rats had significantly lower blood pressure at the ages of 2 and 4 months. However, no significant differences were revealed in the values of both systolic and diastolic pressures between the two groups of animals in the later stages, i.e. at 6 and 8 months of age.

Heart Rate

The resting heart rate of the guanethidine-treated animals was significantly lower than in the age-matched controls at the age of 2 months (Figure 3A). However, values measured at the ages of 4, 6 and 8 months did not differ between the two groups of animals. Cardiac sympathetic nervous tone was estimated by measuring of the negative chronotropic effect of the β-adrenergic receptor antagonist metipranolol. Because of reciprocal interactions between the two branches of the autonomic nervous system, the net effect of metipranolol was tested after previous administration of the muscarinic receptor antagonist atropine. As shown in Figure 3B, metipranolol treatment after atropine administration led to a decrease in the heart rate that was significantly smaller in sympathectomized rats at all time points studied.

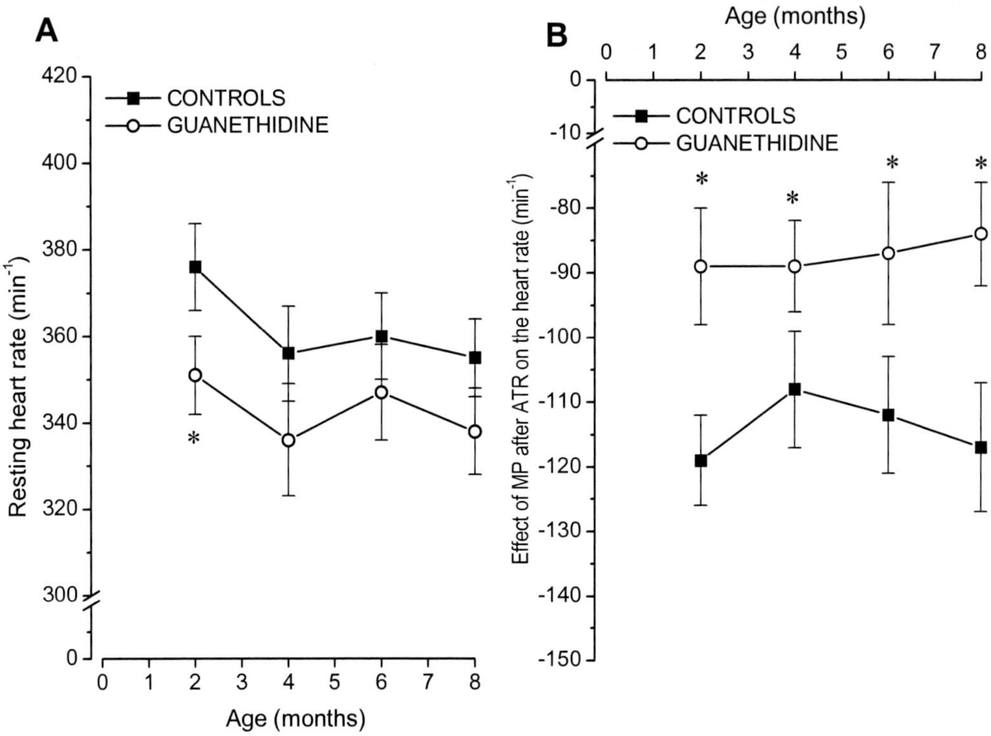

Figure 3A: The resting heart rate in control rats (squares; n = 8) and animals after guanethidine-induced sympathectomy (circles, n = 8) at the ages of 2, 4, 6, and 8 months. B: The effect of metipranolol (MP; 2 mg/kg, s.c) after atropine pretreatment (ATR; 4 mg/kg, s.c.) on the heart rate in control (squares; n = 8) and guanethidine-treated rats (circles; n = 8) at the ages of 2, 4, 6, and 8 months. Data are shown as mean ± SEM. *$p < 0.05$, compared to the respective control value.

Catecholamine Concentrations

To verify the effectivity of the chemical sympathectomy, norepinephrine concentrations were determined in all heart compartments at the ages of 4 and 8 months. The absolute values of norepinephrine levels in the heart compartments of 4-month-old control rats were 936.2 ± 52.0, 787.5 ± 39.3, 585.6 ± 48.9 and 510.6 ± 87.1 ng/g tissue wet weight in the right atria, left atria and free walls of the right and left ventricles, respectively, and they did not change significantly with the age of animals. In the sympathectomized rats at the age of 4 months, norepinephrine concentrations reached 125.9 ± 26.1 and 126.5 ± 27.6 ng/g in the right and left atria, respectively, and even 5.4 ± 2.5 and 2.6 ± 0.3 in the free walls of the right and left ventricles. Interestingly, at the age of 8 months, norepinephrine concentrations in the denervated heart compartments reached significantly higher values compared to those obtained at 4 months of age (right atrium 290 ± 17 ng/g, left atrium 246 ± 19 ng/g, right ventricle 138 ± 11 ng/g and left ventricle 39 ± 5 ng/g – Figure 4).

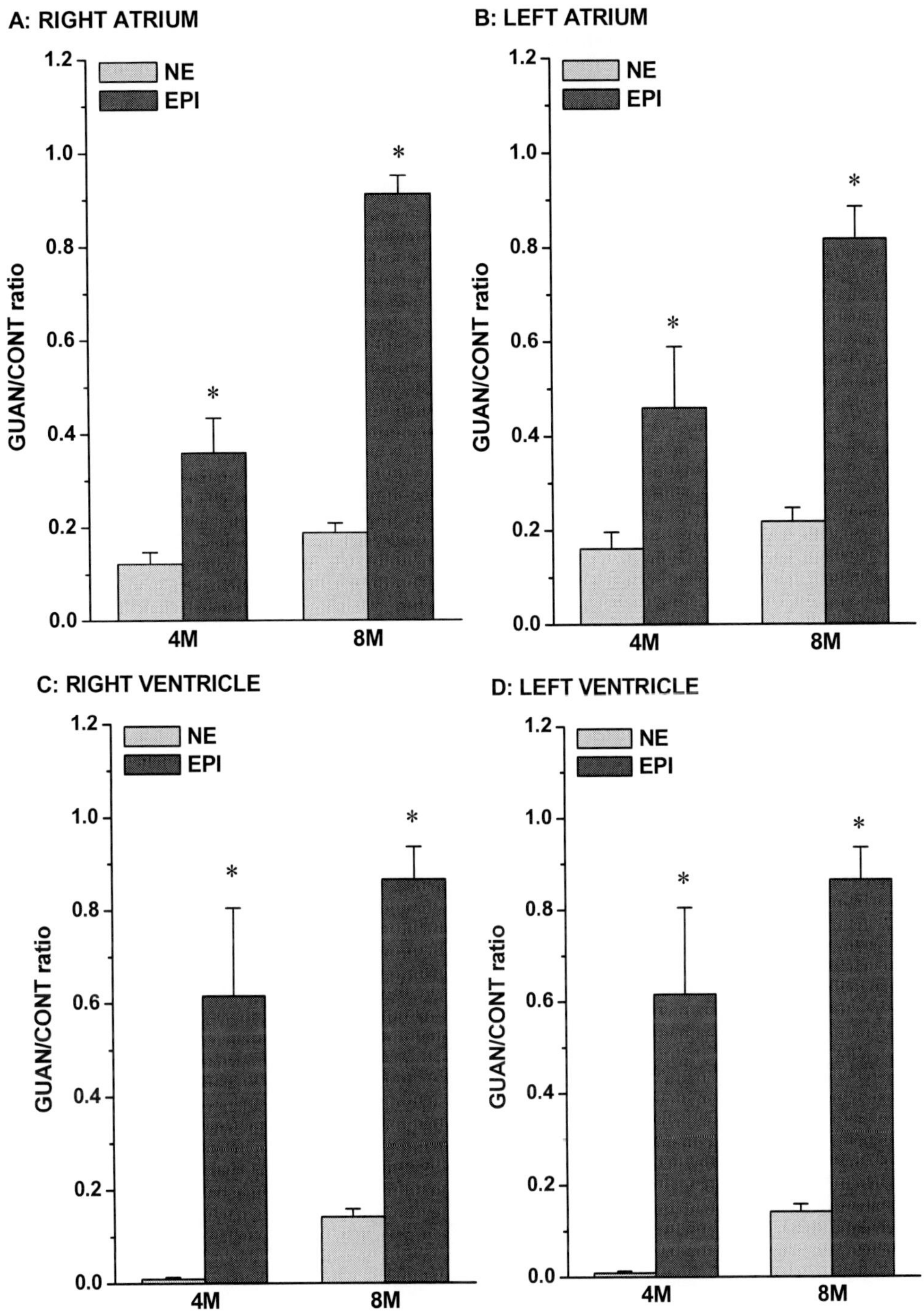

Figure 4. Norepinephrine (NE) and epinephrine (EPI) concentrations in the right atria (A), left atria (B) and free walls of the right and left ventricles (C, D) of 4- and 8-month-old (4M and 8M, respectively) guanethidine-treated rats (GUAN) expressed relatively to the respective control values (CONT). Data are shown as mean ± SEM, n = 6-8 per age category and experimental group. *$p < 0.05$, compared to the respective norepinephrine relative concentration.

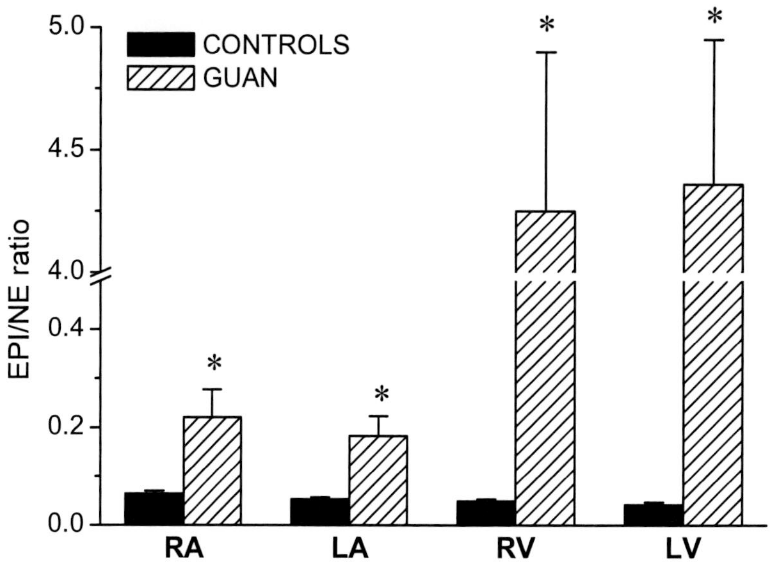

Figure 5. Epinephrine (EPI) to norepinephrine (NE) ratios in the right atria (RA), left atria (LA) and free walls of the right and left ventricles (RV, LV) of 4-month-old guanethidine-treated rats (GUAN) and age-matched control animals (CONTROLS). Data are shown as mean ± SEM, n = 6 per experimental group. *$p < 0.05$, compared to the respective control value.

Epinephrine tissue concentrations of 4-month-old control rats were 63.6 ± 5.9, 41.9 ± 3.5, 28.1 ± 2.3 and 19.6 ± 1.7 ng/g tissue wet weight in the right atria, left atria and free walls of the right and left ventricles, respectively. Since the catecholamines concentrations were determined simultaneously, epinephrine to norepinephrine ratios could be precisely calculated for each sample. In the control heart compartments, these ratios ranged between 0.042 ± 0.004 (left ventricle at the age of 4 months) and 0.08 ± 0.007 (left atrium at the age of 8 months) and they did not significantly differ among individual heart compartments. However, in the denervated hearts, epinephrine concentrations were reduced to much lesser extent than norepinephrine levels at the age of 4 months and they even did not differ from the control levels at the age of 8 months (Figure 4). Epinephrine to norepinephrine ratios significantly increased in the guanethidine-treated rats compared to controls at both ages studied (Figure 5 for 4-month-old rats).

Norepinephrine and Epinephrine Release from the Heart Atria

In the control experiment (Figure 1B), basal release of norepinephrine from the control atria was 22 ± 3 pg/g/min and it was significantly enhanced by depolarization (high KCl; 119 ± 11 pg/g/min). Norepinephrine release measured in the B1 fraction was comparable to that measured in B2 fraction (24 ± 3 pg/g/min). Similarly, norepinephrine outflows in S1 and S2 fractions were not significantly different. As expected, tyramine and desipramine enhanced both basal and KCl-stimulated norepinephrine release from the control atria (Figures 6 and 7). Also, dibutyryl cAMP exerted stimulatory effect on norepinephrine release (Figure 8).

Epinephrine release from the control atria was significantly lower than norepinephrine release and it even fell below the detection limit of the RIA method in some samples measuring the basal outflow. However, stimulated (high KCl) epinephrine release from the control atrial preparations was significantly higher then the basal output. The respective values of epinephrine release in B1, S1, B2, and S2 fractions were 6 ± 0.7, 11 ± 2, 4 ± 0.8 and 10 ± 1 pg/g/min. In the control atria, the general pattern of epinephrine release was similar to norepinephrine output, being stimulated by high K^+ concentration, tyramine, desipramine, and cAMP (Figures 6-8).

Basal release of norepinephrine from the sympathectomized atria was significantly lower than that from the control preparations (8 ± 1 pg/g/min) and it was not enhanced by depolarization. However, tyramine, desipramine and cAMP significantly increased the norepinephrine outflow from the denervated atria (Figures 6, 7, 8).

Epinephrine release from the sympathectomized atria had completely different pattern than norepinephrine release (Figures 6-8). The absolute value of basal epinephrine output did not significantly differ from the control preparations being 6 ± 1 pg/g/min; however it was significantly higher in the presence of dibutyryl cAMP (Figure 8). Depolarization, tyramine and desipramine did not affect the epinephrine release from the denervated atria (Figures 6 and 7).

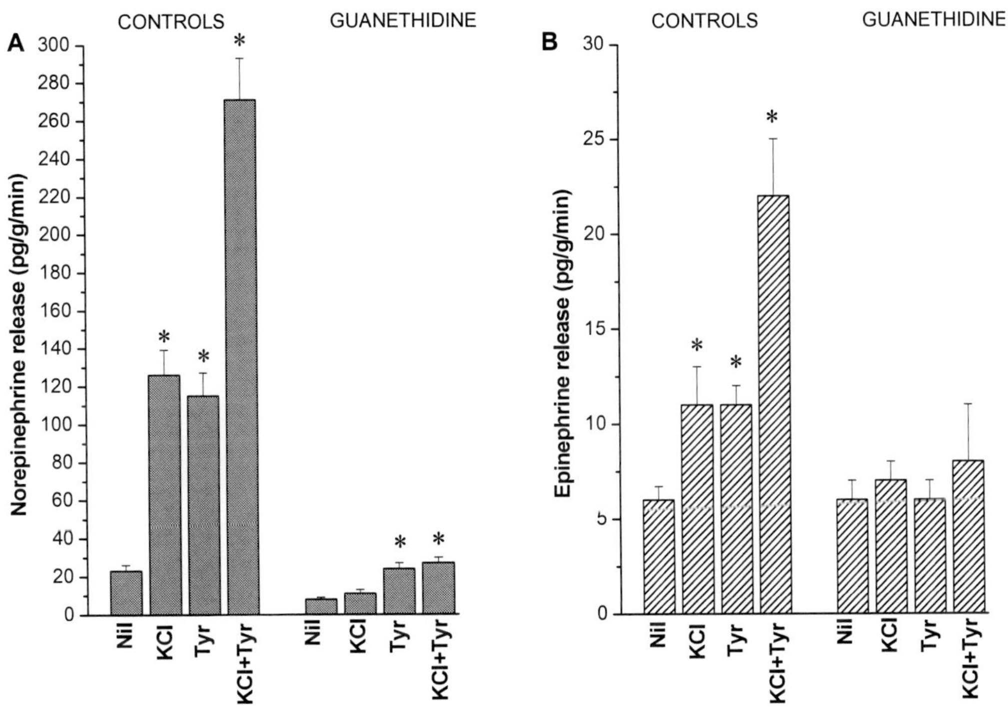

Figure 6. The effect of depolarization (KCl), tyramine (Tyr), and depolarization + tyramine (KCl+Tyr) on norepinephrine (A) and epinephrine (B) release from the control (CONTROLS) and sympathectomized atria (GUANETHIDINE). The results are expressed in pg/g/min as mean ± SEM, n = 4-6. *$p<0.05$, compared to the basal catecholamine outflow (Nil).

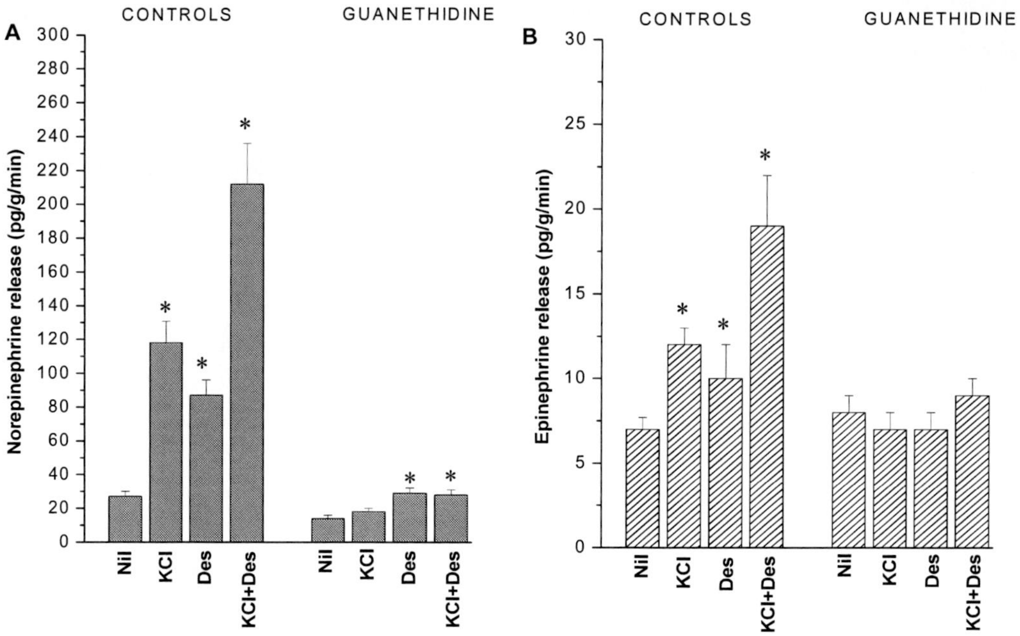

Figure 7. The effect of depolarization (KCl), desipramine (Des), and depolarization + desipramine (KCl+Des) on norepinephrine (A) and epinephrine (B) release from the control (CONTROLS) and sympathectomized atria (GUANETHIDINE). The results are expressed in pg/g/min as mean ± SEM, n = 4-6. *$p<0.05$, compared to the basal catecholamine outflow (Nil).

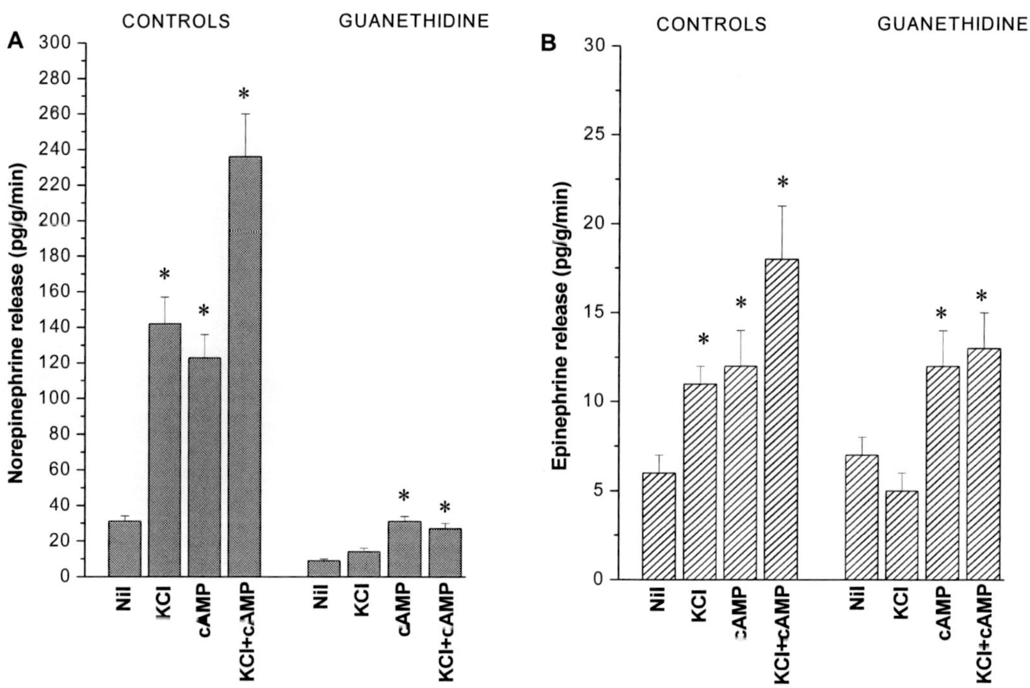

Figure 8. The effect of depolarization (KCl), dibutyryl cAMP (cAMP), and depolarization + dibutyryl cAMP (KCl+cAMP) on norepinephrine (A) and epinephrine (B) release from the control (CONTROLS) and sympathectomized atria (GUANETHIDINE). The results are expressed in pg/g/min as mean ± SEM, n = 4-6. *$p<0.05$, compared to the basal catecholamine outflow (Nil).

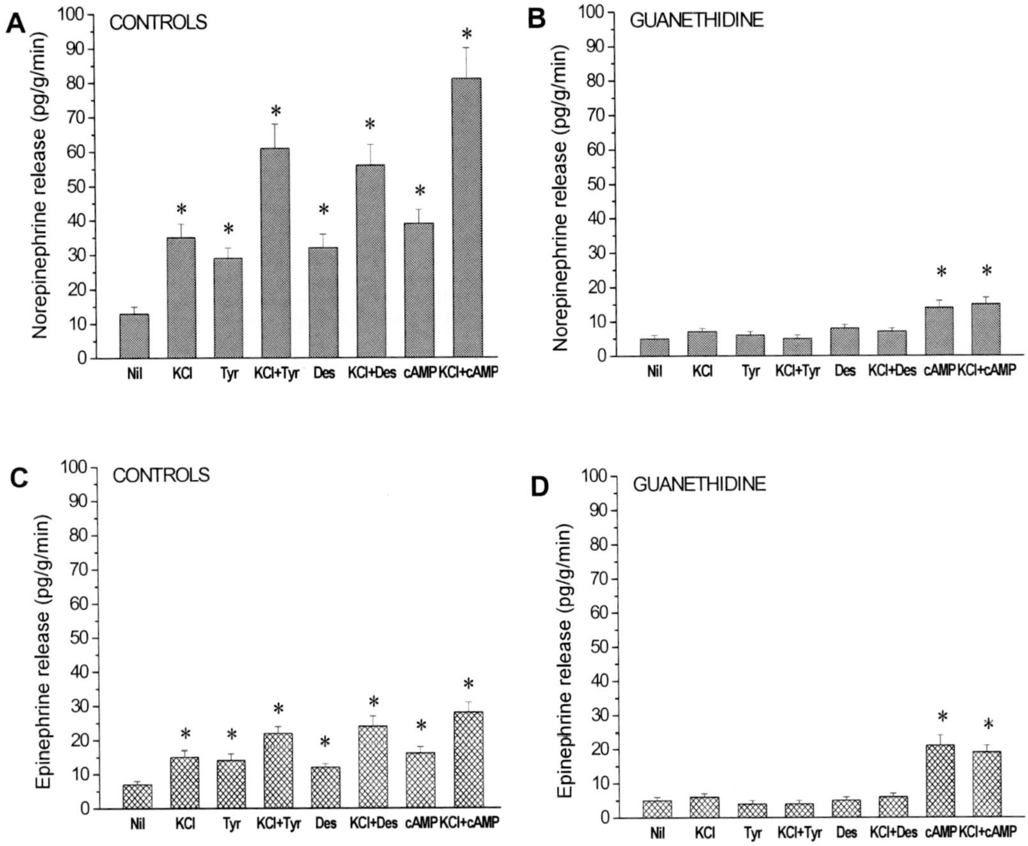

Figure 9. The effect of depolarization (KCl), tyramine (Tyr), depolarization + tyramine (KCl+Tyr), desipramine (Des), depolarization + desipramine (KCl+Des), dibutyryl cAMP (cAMP), and depolarization + dibutyryl cAMP (KCl+cAMP) on norepinephrine (A, B) and epinephrine (C, D) release from the control (CONTROLS) and sympathectomized ventricles (GUANETHIDINE). The results are expressed in pg/g/min as mean ± SEM, n = 4-6. *$p<0.05$, compared to the basal catecholamine outflow (Nil).

Norepinephrine and Epinephrine Release from the Left Ventricles

The difference in norepinephrine and epinephrine release between the control and sympathectomized preparations was even more marked in the left ventricles than in the atria.

In the control left ventricles, both catecholamines outputs were stimulated by depolarization, tyramine, desipramine and cAMP (Figure 9A, C). In contrast, in the denervated preparations, high K^+ concentration, tyramine and desipramine had no effect on both catecholamines outflows. Dibutyryl cAMP significantly enhanced norepinephrine and epinephrine releases in the sympathectomized left ventricles (Figure 9B, D).

Conclusion

In this chapter, we report the results of experiments dealing with differential impact of chemical sympathectomy on epinephrine and norepinephrine concentrations and releases in the rat heart compartments. Administration of guanethidine lasting three postnatal weeks induced an almost complete reduction in norepinephrine concentrations in the heart ventricles of rats at the age of 4 months. The impact of neonatal guanethidine administration on norepinephrine concentrations in the atria was slightly less pronounced, probably reflecting localization of norepinephrine in the intrinsic ganglion neurons and/or chromaffin cells located in the atria, but not in the ventricles [10, 11]. However, at the age of 8 months, norepinephrine concentrations in the denervated heart compartments reached significantly higher values compared to those obtained at 4 months of age, suggesting either partial reinnervation by the noradrenergic fibers or compensatory upregulation of extraneuronal norepinephrine stores. The resting heart rate and blood pressure that were significantly decreased in the sympathectomized animals at the age of 2 or 2 and 4 months, respectively, returned to values not differing from controls later, thus indicating adaptation of the cardiovascular system to the chemical ablation of the sympathetic nerves. However, these putative compensatory changes cannot be straightforwardly attributed to the relative increase in the cardiac norepinephrine content, since the negative chronotropic response to the systemic administration of β-adrenergic antagonist metipranolol remained significantly decreased till the age of 8 months.

The impact of chemical sympathectomy on cardiac epinephrine levels was different: at the age of 4 months, epinephrine concentrations reached ~60% and ~40% of the control values in the atria and ventricles, respectively. Tissue epinephrine levels even did not differ from control values at the age of 8 months. Interestingly, the epinephrine-to-norepinephrine ratios were inversed in the ventricles of 4-month-old sympathectomized rats; clearly suggesting differential cellular origin of the two catecholamines.

The potential sources of cardiac catecholamines in the chronically denervated rats were addressed in the release experiments, where both catecholamines concentrations were measured simultaneously in the perfusates of the control and denervated atrial and left ventricular slices. Norepinephrine release from the postganglionic sympathetic fibers in the mammalian heart has been extensively studied. The release of the neurotransmitter is initiated by a depolarization-induced inward transport of calcium ions to the terminal that is followed by migration of synaptic vesicles towards the neuronal membrane and by exocytosis. The released catecholamine is then removed from the synaptic cleft, particularly by re-uptake of the transmitter into nerve terminals by an active carrier mechanism linked to Na^+-K^+ ATPase [19]. Another mechanism of norepinephrine release from the nerve terminals is mediated by the bi-directional neuronal carrier that normally transports norepinephrine back into the cell. The outward carrier-mediated transport may be induced by at least two mechanisms: by a decrease of the Na^+ concentration gradient across the neuronal membrane or by an increased cytosolic norepinephrine level [20-22]. The neuronal carrier blocker desipramine inhibits the transport of norepinephrine in either direction [22]. Tyramine, a substrate of norepinephrine transporter is taken up into the sympathetic nerve endings and replaces norepinephrine in the synaptic vesicles thus inducing norepinephrine release [20]. Hence, in the reported experiments, we used the interventions that stimulate norepinephrine release either by exocytosis (depolarization of the tissue with high K^+ concentration in the superfusion fluid) or by interference with the uptake mechanism (tyramine and desipramine). In addition, the effect of dibutyryl cAMP was tested due to its documented stimulatory effect on TH activity and norepinephrine turnover in the rat heart [23, 24].

As expected, norepinephrine release from the control heart compartments was stimulated by depolarization, tyramine, desipramine and cAMP. Epinephrine release from the control preparations, although significantly lower in the absolute values, followed the same pattern. In contrast, both catecholamines outflows from the denervated atria and ventricles were not stimulated by depolarization, but were significantly enhanced by cAMP. This finding suggests that cAMP-induced release was not mediated by exocytotic mechanism, since the KCl-induced release of norepinephrine in the rat heart has been repeatedly reported to be calcium-dependent [25, 26].

Drugs interfering with the neuronal uptake, i.e. tyramine and desipramine had differential effect on norepinephrine and epinephrine releases in the denervated atria and ventricles: whereas norepinephrine outflow from the atria was stimulated by both drugs, epinephrine output was not affected at all. In the ventricles, both catecholamines releases were not influenced by tyramine or desipramine. These findings indicate that the putative source cells for epinephrine release from the denervated heart are not equipped with norepinephrine transporter. Besides the sympathetic nerve endings, norepinephrine transporter is expressed in ICA cells [13] and some data indicate that intrinsic cardiac ganglia and catecholaminergic SIF cells also display immunoreactivity to the transporter [27]. In contrast, mRNA for neuronal norepinephrine transporter was not detected in the rat left ventricles [28], suggesting that cardiomyocytes do not display this protein.

Numerous morphological studies indicated that neonatal guanethidine administration leads to permanent loss of the sympathetic neurons in the paravertebral ganglia [29], thus implying that the time-dependent increase in norepinephrine levels in the denervated heart could arise either from the intrinsic cardiac neurons or that the catecholamines stores are replenished from extraneuronal sources. Our data indicate that in the denervated heart, catecholamines could be released, at least in part, from cardiomyocytes. This conclusion is based upon several additional data: 1. PNMT mRNA expression was demonstrated in the right ventricular samples of the transplanted human heart before reinnervation [30]. 2. PNMT immunoreactivity was revealed in the isolated working cardiomyocytes [31]. 3. Chemical sympathectomy with 6-hydroxydopamine increases cardiac PNMT levels [32]. 4. The epinephrine/norepinephrine content and release ratios of ICA cells were reported to be 1/16 and 1/7.5, respectively [12]. In our experiments on sympathectomized heart compartments, epinephrine/norepinephrine content ratios ranged between 1/2.8 in the atria and 1/1.1 in the left ventricles of 8-month-old guanethidine-treated rats. Also, epinephrine/norepinephrine release ratios calculated for basal catecholamine releases were 1/1.3 and 1/1 in the denervated atria and left ventricles, respectively. In addition, sympathectomized preparations were not sensitive to tyramine and desipramine, substances interfering with norepinephrine transporter that is expressed in the ICA cells [13]. These results make the significant contribution of ICA cells to both catecholamines content and release in the sympathectomized heart compartments unlikely.

Taken together, our results provide further evidence of norepinephrine and epinephrine signaling systems independent of the sympathetic innervation in the mammalian heart. Catecholamine release from the non-neuronal sources might help to maintain cardiac function in the absence of sympathetic innervation. Our data also indicate that the denervated left ventricles that are devoid of the intracardiac ganglia may serve as more suitable model to study extraneuronal catecholamine signaling pathways than isolated atria or the whole heart.

Acknowledgements

The present study was supported by the Research project MSM 0021620819: Replacement of and Support to Some Vital Organs awarded by the Ministry of Education, Youth and Sports of the Czech. We thank Kateřina Pícková and Renata Šťastná for excellent technical assistance.

References

[1] Guyton, A; Hall, J. The Autonomic Nervous System and the Adrenal Medulla. In: Guyton A, Hall J: *Textbook of Medical Physiology: Eleventh Edition.* Philadephia, PA: Elsevier Saunders; 2006, 748–756.

[2] Johansson, M; Rundqvist, B; Eisenhofer, G; Friberg, P. Cardiorenal epinephrine kinetics: evidence for neuronal release in the human heart. *Am J Physiol,* 1997, 273, H2178-H2185.

[3] Caramona, MM; Soares da Silva, P. The effects of chemical sympathectomy on dopamine, noradrenaline and adrenaline content in some peripheral tissues. *Br J Pharmacol,* 1985, 86, 351-356.

[4] Villanueva, I; Piñón, M; Quevedo Corona, L; Martínez Olivares; R, Racotta, R. Epinephrine and dopamine colocalization with norepinephrine in various peripheral tissues: guanethidine effects. *Life Sci,* 2003, 73, 1645-1653.

[5] Pendleton, RG; Gessner, G; Sawyer, J. Studies on the distribution of phenylethanolamine N-methyltransferase and epinephrine in the rat. *Res Commun Chem Pathol Pharmacol,* 1978, 21, 315-325.

[6] Hertting, G; Axelrod, J; Kopin, IJ; Whitby, LG. Lack of uptake of catecholamines after chronic denervation of sympathetic nerves. *Nature,* 1961, 7, 189, 66.

[7] Smith, FM; McGuirt, AS; Leger, J; Armour, JA; Ardell, JL. Effects of chronic cardiac decentralization on functional properties of canine intracardiac neurons in vitro. *Am J Physiol Regul Integr Comp Physiol,* 2001, 281, R1474-R1482.

[8] Armour, JA; Collier, K; Kember, G; Ardell, JL. Differential selectivity of cardiac neurons in separate intrathoracic autonomic ganglia. *Am J Physiol Regulatory Integrative Comp Physiol,* 1998, 274, R939–R949.

[9] Slavikova, J; Kuncova, J; Reischig, J; Dvorakova, M. Catecholaminergic neurons in the rat intrinsic cardiac nervous system. *Neurochem Res,* 2003, 28, 593-598.

[10] Pardini, BJ; Patel, KP; Schmid, PG; Lund, DD. Location, distribution and projections of intracardiac ganglion cells in the rat. *J Auton Nerv Syst,* 1987, 20, 91-101.

[11] Batulevicius, D; Pauziene, N; Pauza, DH. Topographic morphology and age-related analysis of the neuronal number of the rat intracardiac nerve plexus. *Ann Anat,* 2003, 185, 449-459.

[12] Huang, MH; Friend, DS; Sunday, ME; Singh, K; Haley, K; Austen, KF; Kelly, RA; Smith, TW. An intrinsic adrenergic system in mammalian heart. *J Clin Invest,* 1996, 98, 1298-1303.

[13] Huang, MH; Bahl, JJ; Wu, Y; Hu, F; Larson, DF; Roeske, WR; Ewy, GA. Neuroendocrine properties of intrinsic cardiac adrenergic cells in fetal rat heart. *Am J Physiol Heart Circ Physiol,* 2005, 288, H497-H503.

[14] Tillinger, A; Bruderova, V; Kubovcakova, L; Zeman, M; Kopacek, J; Novakova, M; Kvetnansky, R; Krizanova, O. Gene expression of the phenylethanolamine N-methyltransferase is differently modulated in cardiac atria and ventricles. Gen *Physiol Biophys,* 2006, 25, 355-364.

[15] Krizanová, O; Micutková, L; Jeloková, J; Filipenko, M; Sabban, E; Kvetnanský, R. Existence of cardiac PNMT mRNA in adult rats: elevation by stress in a glucocorticoid-dependent manner. *Am J Physiol Heart Circ Physiol,* 2001, 281, H1372-H1379.

[16] Kummer, W; Addicks K; Heym, C. Heterogeneity of supracardiac paraganglia. *J Auton Nerv Syst,* 1986, Suppl, 289-293.

[17] Picklo, MJ. Methods of sympathetic degeneration and alteration. *J Auton Nerv Syst,* 1997, 62, 111-125.

[18] Johnson, EM Jr; O'Brien, F; Werbitt, R. Modification and characterization of the permanent sympathectomy produced by the administration of guanethidine to newborn rats. *Eur J Pharmacol,* 1976, 1: 45-54.

[19] Nedergaard, OA. Catecholamines: Regulation, release and inactivation. *Pharm Tox Suppl,* 1988, 63, 5-8.

[20] Langeloh, A; Bönisch, H; Trendelenburg, U. The mechanism of the ^{3}H-noradrenaline releasing effect of various substrates of uptake1: multifactorial induction of outward transport. *Naunyn Schmiedebergs Arch Pharmacol,* 1987, 336, 602-610.

[21] Trendelenburg, U. Carrier-mediated outward transport of noradrenaline from adrenergic varicosities. *Pol J Pharmacol Pharm,* 1990, 42, 515-520.

[22] Levi, G; Raiteri, M. Carrier-mediated release of neurotransmitters. *Trends Neurosci,* 1993, 16, 415-419.

[23] Milanés, MV; Fuente, T; Laorden, ML. Catecholaminergic activity and 3',5'-cyclic adenosine monophosphate levels in heart right ventricle after naloxone induced withdrawal. *Naunyn Schmiedebergs Arch Pharmacol,* 2000, 361, 61-66.

[24] González-Cuello, A; Milanés, MV; Laorden, ML. Increase of tyrosine hydroxylase levels and activity during morphine withdrawal in the heart. *Eur J Pharmacol,* 2004, 506, 119-128.

[25] Dumont, M; Roy, D; Lemaire, S. Nonexocytotic noradrenaline release from rat cardiac synaptosomal-mitochondrial fractions. *J Cardiovasc Pharmacol,* 1997, 30, 302-308.

[26] Kuncová, J; Slavíková, J; Svíglerová, J. Norepinephrine release in the heart atria of diabetic rats. *Gen Physiol Biophys,* 2003, 22, 397-410.

[27] Slavíková, J; Pfeil, U; Paddenberg, R; Kummer, W; Švíglerová, J; Chottová-Dvořáková, M; Kuncová, J. Dopaminergic regulatory system in the rat heart atria. *Physiol Res,* 2007, 56, 31P.

[28] Li, H; Ma, SK; Hu, XP; Zhang, GY; Fei, J. Norepinephrine transporter (NET) is expressed in cardiac sympathetic ganglia of adult rat. *Cell Res,* 2001, 11, 317-320.

[29] Johnson, EM; Manning, PT. Guanethidine-induced destruction of sympathetic neurons. *Int Rev Neurobiol,* 1984, 25, 1–37.

[30] Goncalvesova, E; Krizanova, O; Micutkova, L; Mravec, B; Ksinantova, L; Fabian, J; Kvetnansky, R. Phenylethanolamine N-methyltransferase gene expression in transplanted human heart. *Transplant Proc,* 2005, 37, 1340-1342.

[31] Krizanova, O; Myslivecek, J; Tillinger, A; Jurkovicova, D; Kubovcakova, L. Adrenergic and calcium modulation of the heart in stress: from molecular biology to function. *Stress,* 2007, 10, 173-184.

[32] Elayan, HH; Kennedy, BP; Ziegler, MG. Cardiac atria and ventricles contain different inducible adrenaline synthesising enzymes. *Cardiovasc Res,* 1990, 24, 53-56.

Index

A

B

C

D

E

F

G

H

I

N

Q

R

S

T

U

V

W

X

Y